OUR MISSION

The mission of *Bridging The Gap Foundation* is to improve reproductive health and contraceptive decision making of women and men by providing up-to-date educational resources to the health care providers of tomorrow.

OUR VISION

Our vision is to provide educational resources to the health care providers of tomorrow to help ensure informed choices, better service, access, happier and more successful contraceptors, competent clinicians, fewer unintended pregnancies and disease prevention.

W9-COS-040

www.managingcontraception.com

COPYRIGHT INFORMATION

DISCLAIMER

The authors remind the readers that this book is intended to educate health care providers, not to guide individual therapy. The authors advise a person with a particular problem to consult a primary-care clinician or a specialist in obstetrics, gynecology, or urology (depending on the problem or the contraceptive) as well as the product package insert and other references before diagnosing, managing, or treating the problem. Under no circumstances should the reader use this handbook in lieu of or to override the judgment of the treating clinician. The order in which diagnostic or therapeutic measures appear in this text is not necessarily the order that clinicians *should* follow in each case. The authors and staff are not liable for errors or omissions.

Fourth Edition 2001-2002
ISBN 0-9671939-5-8
Printed in the United States of America
The Bridging the Gap Foundation

On 164 pages, we cannot possibly provide you with all the information you might want or need about contraception. Many of the questions clinicians ask are answered in the textbook *Contraceptive Technology* or in detail on our website. Come visit us regularly at:

www.managingcontraception.com

A POCKET GUIDE TO

MANAGING CONTRACEPTION

2001-2002 Edition

Robert A. Hatcher, MD, MPH
Professor of Gynecology and Obstetrics
Emory University School of Medicine

Anita L. Nelson, MD
Professor of Obstetrics and Gynecology
University of California Los Angeles School of Medicine
Harbor-UCLA Medical Center

Miriam Zieman, MD
Assistant Professor of Gynecology and Obstetrics
Emory University School of Medicine

Philip D. Darney, MD, MSc
Professor of Obstetrics, Gynecology and Reproductive Sciences
University of California, San Francisco
San Francisco General Hospital

Mitchell D. Creinin, MD
Associate Professor of Obstetrics, Gynecology and Reproductive Sciences
University of Pittsburgh School of Medicine
Magee-Womens Hospital

Harriet R. Stosur, MD ←
Clinician in Obstetrics and Gynecology, Kaiser Permanente
Portland, Oregon

Technical and Computer Support:
Anna Poyner, Don Bagwell and Max Harrell
Digital Impact Design, Inc, Cornelia, Georgia

Special Thanks: Copies of *A Pocket Guide to Managing Contraception* are being
sent to all medical students in the United States and to residents and faculty in Family
Medicine and in Obstetrics and Gynecology. They are available thanks to the David and
Lucile Packard Foundation and Organon Inc. Thanks to Organon, Parke Davis and Wyeth,
it has also been possible to provide 130,000 copies of this book to nurses, nurse practitioners and nursing students. We are extremely grateful. If you know of a class of medical
students or a group of residents who have not received copies of this book, please notify
us at our website **www.managingcontraception.com** or call 404-373-0530.

The Bridging the Gap Foundation • Tiger, Georgia

Dear Colleagues and Friends:

Finally, there are four new methods! In October of 2000 the Food and Drug ⟵
Administration approved **Lunelle**, the once-a-month injection, and **Mifiprex** (RU-486 or
mifipristone). Less than 2 months later, in December of 2000, **Mirena**, the levonorgestrel
intrauterine contraceptive was approved. At the end of the year, both the American Medical
Association (AMA) and the American College of Obstetricians and Gynecologists issued
statements favoring pharmacists providing **emergency contraceptive pills** without a
prescription. What an end to the year 2000!

This is the fourth edition of *A Pocket Guide to Managing Contraception*. Thanks to
the generosity of the David and Lucile Packard Foundation, all U.S. medical students and
residents in Obstetrics and Gynecology and Family Medicine programs throughout the
country as well as 80,000 nurses and nursing students and thousands of advanced care
providers received copies of the 1999-2000 edition. Copies of the 2000-2001 book were sent
in September 2000 to 80,000 medical students and residents. Copies of *A Pocket Guide to
Managing Contraception* are provided to nurses at no cost through the National
Association of Nurse Practitioners in Women's Health.

Managing Contraception was developed as a way to put practical information about
birth control and STIs into students' and residents' hands and pockets at the time they need
it. *Contraceptive Technology*, a much longer text, has matured over the course of its 17
editions into a comprehensive reference book that provides essential, readable information
about contraceptive management, reproductive health issues, population dynamics, STIs and
sexuality issues. But even in paperback, its 800-page size limits its portability. To comple-
ment *Contraceptive Technology*, we have created this lightweight, pocket-sized handbook
to meet the immediate needs of medical and nursing students, residents, physicians and
other health care providers. Despite its small print, our target audiences praise the clarity
of flow charts, the practical suggestions, color photos of the various pills, the 1998 CDC STI
Treatment Guidelines, and the small size!

We invite you to put this book to good use and we would appreciate your suggestions and
ideas. Information that has been added since the last edition of *Managing Contraception*
is now easy to find. Look for an arrow! ⟶ or ⟵

Robert A. Hatcher

Robert A. Hatcher, M.D., M.P.H.
Professor of Gynecology and Obstetrics
Emory University School of Medicine
Atlanta, Georgia
President, The Bridging the Gap Foundation

P.S. A new book intended for people who are not medical professionals called *A Personal
Guide to Managing Contraception for Women and Men* complements this handbook.
The *Personal Guide* and the *Pocket Guide* have the same chapters and cover the same
basic information. We hope that you will find the *Personal Guide* helpful for your patients.

We dedicate this edition of

Managing Contraception *to Herbert B. Peterson, MD*
and James D. Shelton, MD

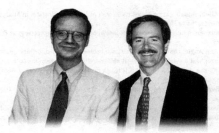

People sometimes wonder about where their tax dollars are going. Bert Peterson and Jim Shelton (and many others, of course) would make you extremely proud of how your money is being spent. They have spent their entire careers in public service, working in an often controversial arena. They have sought to bring high quality contraceptive services to women both in the United States and throughout the world.

Bert Peterson has been at the Centers for Disease Control and Prevention (the CDC) in the Division of Reproductive Health. He has also been a respected, even revered teacher in the Department of Gynecology and Obstetrics at Emory. He is now on a 4 year assignment to the World Health Organization in Geneva. Bert is a quiet, thoughtful, gentle, loving human being. His spirit enriches life for all around him.

Jim Shelton is in charge of population and birth control activities at the U.S. Agency for International Development in Washington, D.C. He has effectively wended0 his way through innumerable political complexities as his agency has provided the funding for most of the international contraceptive activities supported by our government. He continues to see patients in need of contraception. He cares. He cares. He cares. His gentle voice understates his incredible commitment to his life work: the availability on a completely voluntary basis of high quality contraceptive services

Jim Shelton and Bert Peterson's inspiration and hard work led to the World Health Organization Medical Eligibility Criteria for Starting Contraceptive Methods, one of the most successful ventures of the WHO in the field of fertility control (see the Appendix pages A-1 through A-8). Thank you Jim and Bert for lives well lived. The world is a better place for your efforts.

So many have contributed their sensitivity, time, graphics and layout skills, financial support, friendship, encouragement, patience and love in the creation of this *Pocket Guide to Managing Contraception*. This book has been a labor of love—we have tried to condense our thoughts into a format that clinicians and counselors can carry in their pockets, the essential information needed to provide contraceptives. Gems have come to us from many corners. We thank all contributors, including:

- **Jeffrey Allen,** superb, caring breast radiologist at Piedmont Hospital in Atlanta and contributing artist to *MC*
- **Felix Andarsio,** a fine former chief resident in obstetrics and gynecology at Emory University
- **Marcia Ann Angle,** committed international leader in the quest for high quality reproductive health services; at INTRAH at University of North Carolina (UNC), Chapel Hill
- **Anne Atkinson,** training advisor at JHPIEGO; nurse midwifery student at Georgetown; one of tomorrow's leaders
- **Laurie Bazemore,** contraceptive information specialist at the Bridging the Gap Foundation and coordinator of the translation of *MC* into Spanish
- **Audra Bernstein,** first-year curriculum coordinator, Cornell University Medical College
- **Rachel Blankstein,** author of pilot edition of *MC* and Peace Corps volunteer in Niger, Johns Hopkins nursing school student
- **Lynn Borgatta,** medical abortion researcher; OB/GYN faculty at Boston University
- **Stephen Brandt,** research assistant coordinating evaluation of *MC;* has deep reservoirs of concern and caring; and great attention to detail
- **Martha Campbell** and the David and Lucile Packard Foundation, for making *MC* possible
- **Sarah Cates,** medical student at UNC, Chapel Hill. Watch her, world; here comes a great one!
- **Willard Cates,** president, Family Health International, researcher in contraception, STIs, and HIV, and author of *Contraceptive Technology;* cheerleader!
- **Camaryn Chrisman,** medical student at Wake Forest, very helpful in evaluation and distribution of *MC*
- **Sarah Clark,** and staff in the Population Program at the David and Lucile Packard Foundation. Their support of this book from the very start made this effort a reality
- **Sally Faith Dorfman,** director of the Division of Public Health and Education for the Medical Society of New York
- **Susan Eisendrath,** reproductive health initiative director at the American Medical Women's Association; has developed a marvelous reproductive health curriculum for medical schools
- **Erica Frank,** preventionist, environmentalist and associate professor of family and preventive medicine and anatomy at Emory University
- **Meera Garcia,** Emory resident in OB/GYN; one of this world's truly enthusiastic people!
- **Felicia Guest,** AIDS educator, wise observer, and an author of *Contraceptive Technology*
- **John Guillebaud,** professor of family planning and reproductive health at University College London Hospitals and medical director of the Margaret Pyke Center for Study and Training in Family Planning. We thank John for permission to use information from *Contraception Today* (Martin Dunitz Ltd.), London, in *MC*

iii

- **Peter Hatcher**, family practice physician, Multnomah County Health Department, Portland, Oregon; lover of gardening, photography, his family, dogs and a loyal friend
- **Andrew Kaunitz**, professor and assistant chair, OB/GYN department, University of Florida; Health Sciences Center, Jacksonville, Florida
- **Maxine Keel**, administrative assistant at the Emory University Family Planning Program, dreamer, inspiration and friend
- **Monica McGrann**, medical student with indomitable enthusiasm, Texas A&M
- **Radhika Mohan**, University of Washington student ('01), edited pilot edition of *MC* and was photographed for page in this book designed to teach the pill danger signals (on right, page 94)
- **LeRoy Nelson**, remarkable editor of every page of the 2000-2001 book
- **Bert Peterson,** contraceptive research leader at the CDC in Atlanta and at the WHO in Geneva; former gynecology professor at Emory (see dedication on p. ii)
- **Erika Pluhar**, PhD author of *A Personal Guide to Managing Contraception*. Dissertation in human sexuality on mother/daughter communication
- **Malcolm Potts**, perhaps the most creative force in the field of family planning, human sexuality and reproductive health. Students at U.C. Berkely love him.
- **Anna Poyner**, graphic artist who designed every page in this book; Digital Impact Design in Cornelia, Georgia
- **Ida Rastegar**, Emory Medical School student - class of 2002
- **Sharon Schnare**, dreamer, nurse practitioner and nurse midwife consultant and trainer in Seattle; remarkable teacher
- **Tara Shochet**, Research Assistant at the Office of Population Research at Princeton University, who offered so many detailed observations leading to small and large improvements in this book
- **Andrea Tone**, historian in the Department of History, Technology and Society at Georgia Tech, Atlanta; specializing in the history of contraception
- **James Trussell**, an author of *Contraceptive Technology* who developed the failure rates and cost figures used throughout *MC*; champion of emergency contraception
- **Marcel Vekemans**, a family planning specialist from Belgium working at INTRAH whose attention to detail improved this book so much
- **Jane Wamsher**, nurse practitioner at Grady Memorial Hospital in Atlanta; provided practical protocols and creative techniques for using book to teach
- **Ian Weisberg**, Emory Medical School student - class of 2002
- **Lee Warner**, CDC researcher working on STDs and HIV; so much help on the condom chapters
- **Elisa S. Wells**, senior program officer at PATH; emergency contraception expert
- **Anne Zweifel**, fine resident in OB/GYN at UNC, Chapel Hill

ACOG	American College of Obstetricians & Gynecologists	**FAM**	Fertility awareness methods
		FDA	Food and Drug Administration
AIDS	Acquired immunodeficiency syndrome	**FH**	Family History
		FSH	Follicle stimulating hormone
AMA	American Medical Association	**GC**	gonococcus/gonorrhea
ASAP	As soon as possible	**GI**	gastrointestinal
BBT	Basal body temperature	**GnRH**	Gonadotropin-releasing hormone
BCA	Bichloroacetic acid		
BP	Blood Pressure	**HBsAg**	Hepatitis B surface antigen
BV	Bacterial vaginosis	**HBV**	Hepatitis B virus
CDC	Centers for Disease Control and Prevention	**HCG**	Human chorionic gonadotrophin
		HDL	High density lipoprotein
COCs	Combined oral contraceptives (estrogen & progestin)	**HIV**	Human immunodeficiency virus
CMV	Cytomegalovirus	**HPV**	Human papillomavirus
CT	*Contraceptive Technology*	**HRT**	Hormone replacement therapy (estrogen & progestin)
D & C	Dilation and curettage		
DMPA	Depot-medroxyprogesterone acetate (Depo-Provera)	**HSV**	Herpes simplex virus (I or II)
		IM	Intramuscular
DUB	Dysfunctional uterine bleeding	**IPPF**	International Planned Parenthood Federation
DVT	Deep vein thrombosis		
E	Estrogen	**IUD**	Intrauterine device
EC	Emergency contraception	**IUS**	Intrauterine system
ECPs	Emergency contraceptive pills ("morning-after pills")	**IV**	Intravenous
		KOH	Potassium hydroxide
ED	Erectile dysfunction	**LAM**	Lactation amenorrhea method
E$_2$	Estradiol	**LDL**	Low-density lipoprotein
EE	Ethinyl estradiol	**LGV**	Lymphogranuloma venereum
ERT	Estrogen replacement therapy		

v

LH	Luteinizing hormone	**PMS**	Premenstrual syndrome
LMP	Last menstrual period	**po**	Latin: "Per os"; orally
MI	Myocardial infarction	**POCs**	Progestin-only contraceptives
MIS	Misoprostol	**POP**	Progestin-only pill (minipill)
MMPI	Minnesota Multiphasic Personality Inventory	**PP**	Postpartum
MMWR	Mortality and Morbidity Weekly Report	**PPFA**	Planned Parenthood Federation of America
MPA	Medroxyprogesterone acetate	**RR**	Relative risk
MTX	Methotrexate	**Rx**	Treatment
MVA	Manual vacuum aspiration	**SAB**	Spontaneous abortion
NFP	Natural family planning	**STD**	Sexually transmitted disease
NSAID	Nonsteroidal anti-inflammatory drug	**STI**	Sexually transmissible infection
OA	Overeaters Anonymous	**TAB**	Therapeutic abortion
OB/GYN	Obstetrics & Gynecology	**TB**	Tuberculosis
OC	Oral contraceptive	**TCA**	Trichloroacetic acid
OR	Operating Room	**TSS**	Toxic shock syndrome
P	Progesterone	**URI**	Upper respiratory infection
PCOS	Polycystic ovarian syndrome	**UTI**	Urinary tract infection
PE	Pulmonary embolism	**VTE**	Venous thromboembolism
pH	Hydrogen ion concentration	**VVC**	Vulvovaginal candidiasis
PID	Pelvic inflammatory disease	**WHO**	World Health Organization
PLISSIT	Permission giving	**ZDV**	Zidovudine
	Limited information		
	Simple suggestions		
	Intensive		
	Therapy		

Please see form at end of book or call 404-373-0530 to order additional copies of *Managing Contraception*

vi

1. Carry it with you. Arrows are a simple way for you to find the new information in this edition: ➤ or ◄

2. Chapter 35 is taken directly from the 1998 CDC recommended guidelines for the treatment of STIs. These guidelines cover routine cases, pregnancy recommendations, ➤ and more complicated cases (2001 update is coming in 2002-3 edition of *MC*)

3. Color photos of pills will help you to determine the pill your patient is/was on ➤ (see the very end of the book).

4. The pages on the menstrual cycle concisely explain a very complicated series of events. Study pages 1-3 over and over again. Favorite subjects for exams!

5. Algorithms throughout book; several that might help you are on the following pages:
   - Page 108: Choosing a pill
   - Page 109: What to do about breakthrough bleeding or spotting on pills
   - Page 119: What to do if a woman returns late for her Depo-Provera injection

➤ 6. If you know the page number for the 2000-2001 edition, the information in your 2001-2002 book is likely to be on *about* the same page. The order of chapters is unchanged

IMPORTANT PHONE NUMBERS

TOPIC	ORGANIZATION	PHONE NUMBER
Abortion	Abortion Hotline (NAF)	800-772-9100
Abuse/Rape	National Committee to Prevent Child Abuse	(312) 663-3520
	Coalition on Domestic Violence	800-537-2238
	CDC Rape Hotline (RAIN)	800-656-4673
		800-344-7432 Spanish
		800-243-7889
Adoption	Adopt a Special Kid-America	(202) 857-9708
	Adoptive Families of America	(651) 644-5223
Breastfeeding	La Leche League	800-LA-LECHE
Contraception	Planned Parenthood	800-230-7526
	Family Health International	(919) 544-7040
	PPFA	(212) 541-7800
Counseling	Peer Counseling for Gay/Lesbian	800-969-6884
	Peer Listening Line Gay/Lesbian	800-399-7337
	Depression after Delivery	800-944-4773
Emergency contraception	Emergency Contraception Information	888-NOT-2-LATE
		888-PREVEN2
HIV/AIDS	CDC AIDS Hotline	800-342-2437
	CDC National AIDS Clearinghouse	800-458-5231
	AIDS Clinical Trials Information Service	800-874-2572
Pregnancy	Lamaze International	800-368-4404
STIs	Hepatitis B Coalition	(651) 647-9009
	CDC Sexually Transmitted Disease	800-227-8922
	Herpes and HPV Hotline	800-230-6039

SEVERAL KEY POINTS ON MENSTRUAL PHYSIOLOGY:

- **What initiates menses (and the next cycle)** is atrophy of the corpus luteum from the current cycle, leading to a fall in serum estrogen (E) and progesterone (P) levels. Without hormonal support, the endometrium sloughs. This drop in hormonal levels is also detected by the hypothalamus and pituitary, and FSH levels increase to stimulate follicles for the next cycle (see Figures 1.1 and 1.2).

- **Anovulatory cycles in women taking pills are regular** because the pills containing estrogen and progestin stimulate and support the endometrium. When the placebo (sugar) pills are taken the drop in circulating hormone levels causes withdrawal bleeding.

- **The two-cell, two gonadotrophin theory:** LH-stimulated *theca* cells comprise the outer cell layer surrounding the follicle and produce androgens (testosterone and androstenedione). These androgens diffuse toward the inner layer *granulosa* cells where they are converted into estradiol (E_2) by FSH-stimulated aromatase (see Figure 1.3).

- In a developing follicle, *low androgen levels* not only serve as the substrate for FSH-induced aromatization, but also stimulate aromatase activity.

- On the other hand, **high levels of androgens** (an "androgen-rich" environment) lead to inhibition of aromatase activity and to follicular atresia.

- Each woman is born with millions of follicles, most of which undergo atresia before puberty. Hundreds of thousands of other follicles are lost in the preantral stage during the reproductive years. Only about 18-20 follicles each month are recruited by rising FSH levels. Of those 18-20 follicles, usually only one dominant follicle is allowed to ovulate. The dominant follicle starts with adequate (but not excessive) androgen substrate and adequate numbers of FSH receptors.

- FSH levels drop 4-5 days before ovulation as a result of negative feedback from FSH-stimulated production of E_2 and the protein inhibin. The dominant follicle "escapes" the effects of falling FSH levels before ovulation, because it has more granulosa cells, more FSH receptors on each of its granulosa cells, and increased blood flow. Cut off from adequate FSH stimulation, the other follicles undergo atresia.

- Once the other follicles are out of the picture, leaving only the dominant follicle, total production of E_2 and inhibin drops, FSH levels rise again. This induces an outpouring of E_2 from the dominant follicle. When E_2 production is sustained at sufficient levels for more than 100 hours, negative feedback of E_2 on LH reverses into positive feedback. The LH surge occurs, and an oocyte is extruded.

- From the remaining cells, the corpus luteum is formed. Some granulosa cells continue to produce E_2 and inhibins but many join the outer layers of theca cells to produce progesterone (P) and activin. Inhibin selectively suppresses FSH, not LH. The highest levels of inhibin are during the mid-luteal phase, causing FSH levels to be the lowest in the mid-luteal phase. At the end of the cycle (10-14 days after ovulation) if the corpus luteum is not rescued by HCG produced by the implanted trophoblast, the corpus luteum will undergo programmed atresia. Falling E_2, P, and inhibin levels induce the release of FSH to initiate another cycle.

Figure 1.1 Menstrual cycle events – Idealized 28 Day Cycle
[Hatcher RA, et al. *Contraceptive Technology*. 16th ed. New York: Irvington, 1994:41]

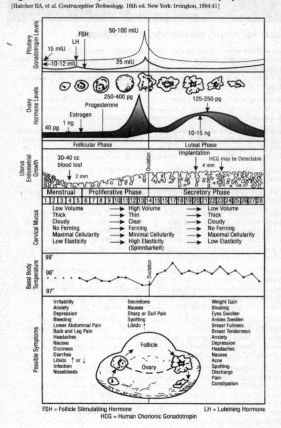

FSH = Follicle Stimulating Hormone   LH = Luteining Hormone
HCG = Human Chorionic Gonadotropin

Figure 1.2 Regulation of the menstrual cycle
[Hatcher RA, et al. *Contraceptive Technology*. 16th ed. New York: Irvington, 1994:40]

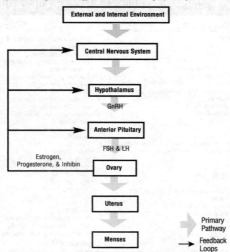

Primary hormone pathways (➡) in the reproductive system are modulated by both negative and positive feedback loops (→). Prostaglandins, secreted by the ovary and by uterine endometrial cells, also play a role in ovulation, and may modulate hypothalamic function as well.

Figure 1.3 The Two-cell, two gonadotrophin theory

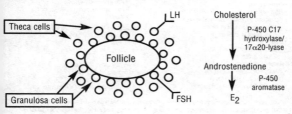

CHAPTER 2
Recommended Screening/Risk Assessment by Age**

AGES 13-18 YEARS

SCREENING
History
- Reason for visit
- Health status: medical, surgical, family
- Dietary/nutrition assessment
- Physical activity
- Use of complementary and alternative medicine
- Tobacco, alcohol, other drug use
- Abuse/neglect
- Sexual practices

Physical Examination
- Height
- Weight
- Blood pressure
- Secondary sexual characteristics (Tanner staging)
- Pelvic examination (yearly when sexually active or by age 18)
- Skin*

LABORATORY TESTS
Periodic
- Pap test (if sexually active or by age 18)

*High-Risk Groups**
- Hemoglobin level assessment
- Bacteriuria testing
- STI testing
- HIV testing
- Genetic testing/counseling
- Rubella titer assessment
- Tuberculosis skin test
- Lipid profile assessment
- Fasting glucose
- Cholesterol testing
- Hepatitis C virus testing
- Colorectal cancer screening

EVALUATION AND COUNSELING
Sexuality
- Development
- High-risk behaviors
- Preventing unwanted/unintended pregnancy
    Postponing sexual involvement
    Contraceptive options
- STIs
    Partner selection
    Barrier protection

Fitness and Nutrition
- Dietary/nutritional assessment
  (including eating disorders)
- Exercise: discussion of program

- Folic acid supplementation (0.4 mg/d)
- Calcium intake

Psychosocial Evaluation
- Interpersonal/family relationships
- Sexual identity
- Personal goal development
- Behavioral/learning disorders
- Abuse/neglect
- Satisfactory school experience
- Peer relationships

Cardiovascular Risk Factors
- Family history
- Hypertension
- Dyslipidemia
- Obesity
- Diabetes mellitus

Health/Risk Behaviors
- *Hygiene (including dental); fluoride
  supplementation*
- Injury prevention
    - Safety belts and helmets
    - Recreational hazards
    - Firearms
    - Hearing
- Skin exposure to ultraviolet rays
- Suicide: depressive symptoms
- Tobacco, alcohol, other drug use

IMMUNIZATIONS
Periodic
- Tetanus-diphtheria booster (once between
  ages 11 and 16 years)
- Hepatitis B vaccine (one series for those not
  previously immunized)

*High-Risk Groups**
- Influenza vaccine
- Hepatitis A vaccine
- Pneumococcal vaccine
- Measles, mumps, rubella vaccine
- Varicella vaccine

Leading Causes of Death:
- Motor vehicle accidents
- Homicide
- Suicide
- Cancer
- All other accidents and adverse effects
- Diseases of the heart
- Congenital anomalies
- Chronic obstructive pulmonary diseases

**Many organizations have screening guidelines. These are reprinted with permission from the American
College of Obstetricians and Gynecologists from *Precis, Primary and Preventive Care: An Update in
Obstetrics and Gynecology.* 1998. Revised December, 2000; ACOG Committee Opinion No 246.

Leading Causes of Morbidity:

- Acne
- Asthma
- Chlamydia
- Depression
- Dermatitis
- Headaches
- Infective, viral, and parasitic diseases
- Influenza
- Injuries
- Nose, throat, ear and upper respiratory infections
- Sexual assault
- Sexually transmitted deseases
- Urinary tract infections

* Please see page 8 for High-Risk Factors

AGES 19-39 YEARS

SCREENING

History
- Reason for visit
- Health status: medical, surgical, family
- Dietary/nutrition assessment
- Physical activity
- Use of complementary and alternative medicine
- Tobacco, alcohol, other drug use
- Abuse/neglect
- Sexual practices
- Urinary and fecal incontinence

Physical Examination
- Height
- Weight
- Blood pressure
- Neck, adenopathy, thyroid
- Breasts
- Abdomen
- Pelvic examination
- Skin*

LABORATORY TESTING

Periodic
- Pap test (physician and patient discretion after three consecutive normal tests if low risk)

For High-Risk Groups*
- Hemoglobin level assessment
- Bacteriuria testing
- Mammography
- Fasting glucose test
- Cholesterol testing
- STI testing
- HIV testing
- Genetic testing/counseling
- Rubella titer assessment
- Tuberculosis skin testing
- Lipid profile assessment
- Thyroid-stimulating hormone testing
- Hepatitis C virus testing
- Colorectal cancer screening

EVALUATION AND COUNSELING

Sexuality
- High-risk behaviors
- Contraceptive options for prevention of unwanted pregnancy
- Preconceptional and genetic counseling for desired pregnancy
- STIs
    Partner selection
    Barrier protection
- Sexual function

Fitness and Nutrition
- Dietary/nutritional assessment
- Exercise: discussion of program
- Folic acid supplementation (0.4 mg/d)
- Calcium intake

Psychosocial Evaluation
- Interpersonal/family relationships
- Domestic violence
- Work satisfaction
- Lifestyle/stress
- Sleep disorders

Cardiovascular Risk Factors
- Family history
- Hypertension
- Dyslipidosis
- Obesity
- Diabetes mellitus
- Lifestyle

Health/Risk Behaviors
- Hygiene (including dental)
- Injury prevention
    - Safety belts and helmets
    - Occupational hazards
    - Recreational hazards
    - Firearms
    - Hearing
- Breast self-examination
- Chemoprophylaxis for breast cancer (for high-risk women ages 35 years or older)
- Skin exposure to ultraviolet rays
- Suicide: depressive symptoms
- Tobacco, alcohol, other drug use

IMMUNIZATIONS

Periodic
- Tetanus-diphtheria booster (every 10 years)

For High-Risk Factors*
- Measles, mumps, rubella vaccine
- Hepatitis A vaccine
- Hepatitis B vaccine
- Influenza vaccine
- Pneumococcal vaccine
- Varicella vaccine

* Please see page 9 for High-Risk Factors

Leading Causes of Death:
- Accidents and adverse effects
- Cancer
- HIV infection
- Diseases of the heart
- Homicide
- Suicide
- Cerebrovascular disease
- Chronic liver disease and cirrhosis

Leading Causes of Morbidity:
- Asthma
- Back symptoms
- Breast disease
- Deformity or orthopedic impairment
- Depression
- Diabetes
- Gynecologic disorders
- Headache/migraines
- Hypertension
- Infective, viral, and parasitic diseases
- Influenza
- Injuries
- Nose, throat, ear, and upper respiratory infections
- Sexual assault/domestic violence
- Sexually transmitted diseases
- Skin rash/dermatitis
- Substance abuse
- Urinary tract infections
- Vaginitis

AGES 40–64 YEARS

SCREENING
History
- Reason for visit
- Health status: medical, surgical, family
- Dietary/nutrition assessment
- Physical activity
- Use of complementary and alternative medicine
- Tobacco, alcohol, other drug use
- Abuse/neglect
- Sexual practices
- Urinary and fecal incontinence

Physical Examination
- Height
- Weight
- Blood pressure
- Oral cavity
- Neck: adenopathy, thyroid
- Breasts, axillae
- Abdomen
- Pelvic examination
- Skin*

LABORATORY TESTING
Periodic
- Pap test (physician and patient discretion after three consecutive normal tests if low risk)

- Mammography (every 1-2 years until age 50, yearly beginning at age 50)
- Cholesterol (every 5 yrs beginning at age 45)
- Yearly fecal occult blood testing plus flexible sigmoidoscopy every 5 years or colonoscopy every 10 years or double contrast barium enema (DCBE) every 5-10 years, with digital rectal examination performed at the time of each screening sigmoidoscopy, colonoscopy, or DCBE (beginning at age 50)
- Fasting glucose testing (every 3 years after age 45)

High-Risk Groups*
- Hemoglobin level assessment
- Bacteriuria testing
- Fasting glucose testing
- STI testing
- HIV testing
- Tuberculosis skin testing
- Lipid profile assessment
- Thyroid-stimulating hormone testing
- Hepatitis C virus testing
- Colorectal cancer screening

EVALUATION AND COUNSELING
Sexuality+
- High-risk behaviors
- Contraceptive options for prevention of unwanted pregnancy
- STIs
  - Partner selection
  - Barrier protection
- Sexual function

Fitness and Nutrition
- Dietary/nutrition assessment
- Exercise: discussion of program
- Folic acid supplementation (0.4 mg/d before age 50 years)
- Calcium intake

Psychosocial Evaluation
- Family relationships
- Domestic violence
- Work satisfaction
- Retirement planning
- Lifestyle/stress
- Sleep disorders

Cardiovascular Risk Factors
- Family history
- Hypertension
- Dyslipidemia
- Obesity
- Diabetes mellitus
- Lifestyle

Health/Risk Behaviors
- Hygiene (including dental)
- Hormone replacement therapy
- Injury prevention
  - Safety belts and helmets
  - Occupational hazards

+Preconceptional counseling is appropriate for certain women in this age group.

* Please see page 9 for High Risk Factors.

6

- Recreational hazards
- Sports involvement
- Firearms
- Hearing
- Breast self-examination
- Chemoprophylaxis for breast cancer (for high risk women)
- Skin exposure to ultraviolet rays
- Suicide: depressive symptoms
- Tobacco, alcohol, other drug use

IMMUNIZATIONS
Periodic
- Influenza vaccine (annually beginning at age 50)
- Tetanus-diphtheria booster (every 10 yrs)

High-Risk Groups*
- Measles, mumps, rubella vaccine
- Hepatitis A vaccine
- Hepatitis B vaccine
- Influenza vaccine
- Pneumococcal vaccine
- Varicella vaccine

Leading Causes of Death:
- Cancer
- Diseases of the heart
- Cerebrovascular diseases
- Accidents and adverse effects
- Chronic obstructive pulmonary disease
- Diabetes mellitus
- Chronic liver disease and cirrhosis
- Pneumonia and influenza

Leading Causes of Morbidity:
- Arthritis/osteoarthritis
- Asthma
- Back symptoms
- Breast disease
- Cardiovascular disease
- Carpal tunnel syndrome
- Deformity or orthopedic impairment
- Depression
- Diabetes
- Headache
- Hypertension
- Infective, viral, and parasitic diseases
- Influenza
- Injuries
- Menopause
- Nose, throat, and upper respiratory infections
- Obesity
- Skin conditions/dermatitis
- Substance abuse
- Urinary tract infections
- Urinary tract (other conditions including urinary incontinence)
- Vision impairment

AGE 65 YEARS AND OLDER

SCREENING
History
- Reason for visit
- Health status: medical, surgical, family
- Dietary/nutritional assessment
- Physical activity
- Use of complementary and alternative medicine
- Tobacco, alcohol, other drug use, and concurrent medication use
- Abuse/neglect
- Sexual practices
- Urinary and fecal incontinence

Physical Examination
- Height
- Weight
- Blood pressure
- Oral cavity
- Neck: adenopathy, thyroid
- Breasts, axillae
- Abdomen
- Pelvic examination
- Skin*

LABORATORY TESTING
Periodic
- Pap testing (physician and patient discretion after three consecutive normal tests if low risk)
- Urinalysis
- Mammography
- Cholesterol testing (every 3-5 years before age 75 years)
- Yearly fecal occult blood testing plus flexible sigmoidoscopy every 5 years or colonoscopy every 10 years or double contrast barium enema (DCBE) every 5-10 years, with digital rectal examination performed at the time of each screening sigmoidoscopy, colonoscopy, or DCBE
- Fasting glucose testing (every 3 years)

High-Risk Factors*
- Hemoglobin level assessment
- STI testing
- HIV testing
- Tuberculosis skin testing
- Lipid profile assessment
- Thyroid-stimulating hormone testing
- Hepatitis C virus testing
- Colorectal cancer screening

EVALUATION AND COUNSELING
Sexuality
- Sexual functioning
- Sexual behaviors
- STIs
   Partner selection
   Barrier protection

*Please see page 9 for High Risk Factors

Fitness and Nutrition
- Dietary/nutrition assessment
- Exercise: discussion of program
- Calcium intake

Psychosocial Evaluation
- Neglect/abuse
- Lifestyle/stress
- Depression/sleep disorders
- Family relationships
- Work/retirement satisfaction

Cardiovascular Risk Factors
- Hypertension
- Dyslipidemia
- Obesity
- Diabetes mellitus
- Sedentary lifestyle

Health/Risk Behaviors
- Hygiene (general and dental)
- Hormone replacement therapy
- Injury prevention
  - Safety belts and helmets
  - Prevention of falls
  - Occupational & Recreational hazards
  - Firearms
- Visual acuity/glaucoma
- Hearing
- Breast self-examination
- Chemoprophylaxis for breast cancer (for high risk women)
- Skin exposure to ultraviolet rays
- Suicide: depressive symptoms
- Tobacco, alcohol, other drug use

IMMUNIZATIONS
Periodic
- Tetanus-diphtheria booster (every 10 yrs)
- Influenza vaccine (annually)
- Pnesumococcal vaccine (once)

High-Risk Groups*
- Hepatitis A vaccine
- Hepatitis B vaccine
- Varicella vaccine

Leading Causes of Death:
- Diseases of the heart
- Cancer
- Cerebrovascular diseases
- Chronic obstructive pulmonary diseases
- Pneumonia/influenza
- Diabetes mellitus
- Accidents and adverse effects
- Alzheimer's disease

Leading Causes of Morbidity:
- Arthritis/osteoarthritis
- Back symptoms
- Breast cancer
- Chronic obstructive pulmonary diseases
- Cardiovascular disease
- Deformity or orthopedic impairment
- Degeneration of macula retinae and posterior pole
- Diabetes
- Hearing and vision impairment
- Hypertension
- Hypothyroidism and other thyroid disease
- Influenza
- Nose, throat, and upper respiratory infections
- Osteoporosis
- Skin lesion/dermatoses/dermatitis
- Urinary tract infections
- Urinary tract (other conditions including urinary incontinence)
- Vertigo

INTERVENTIONS FOR HIGH-RISK FACTORS

Intervention	High-Risk Factor
• Bacteriuria testing	Diabetes mellitus
• Cholesterol testing	Familial lipid disorders; family history (FH) of premature coronary heart disease; history of coronary heart disease.
• Colorectal cancer screening	Colorectal cancer or adenomatous polyps in first-degree relative younger than 60 years or in two or more first-degree relatives of any ages; family history of familial adenomatous polyposis or hereditary nonpolyposis colon cancer; history of colorectal cancer, adenomatous polyps, or inflammatory bowel disease
• Fasting glucose test	Obesity; first-degree relative with diabetes mellitus; member of a high risk ethnic population (eg, African American, Hispanic, Native American, Asian, Pacific Islander); have delivered a baby weighing more than 9 lb or history of gestational diabetes mellitus; hypertensive; high-density lipoprotein cholesterol level of at least 35 mg/dL; triglyceride level of at least 250 mg/dL; history of impaired glucose tolerance or impaired fasting glucose
• Fluoride supplementation	Live in area with inadequate water fluoridation (<0.7 ppm)
• Genetic testing/counseling	Exposure to teratogens; considering pregnancy at age 35 or older; patient partner, or family member with history of genetic disorder or birth defect; African, Eastern European Jewish, Mediterranean, or African ancestry
• Hemoglobin level assessment	Caribbean, Latin American, Asian, Mediterranean, or African ancestry; history of excessive menstrual flow
• Hepatitis A vaccination	International travelers; illegal drug users; people who work with nonhuman primates; chronic liver disease; clotting-factor disorders; sex partners of bisexual men; measles, mumps, and rubella nonimmune persons; food-service workers; health-care workers; daycare workers
• Hepatitis B vaccination	Intravenous drug users and their sexual contacts; recipients of clotting factor concentrates; occupational exposure to blood or blood products; patients and workers in dialysis units; persons with chronic renal or hepatic disease; household or sexual contact with hepatitis B virus carriers; history of sexual activity with multiple partners; history of sexual activity with sexually active homosexual or bisexual men; international travelers; residents and staff of institutions for the developmentally disabled and of correctional institutions
• Hepatitis C virus (HCV) testing	History of injecting illegal drugs; recipients of clotting factor concentrates before 1987; chronic (long-term) hemodialysis; persistently abnormal alanine aminotransferase levels; recipient of blood from a donor who later tested positive for HCV infection; recipient of blood or blood-component transfusion or organ transplant before July 1992; occupational percutaneous or mucosal exposure to HCV-positive blood
• Human immunodeficiency virus (HIV) testing	Seeking treatment for STIs; drug use by injection; history of prostitution; past or present sexual partner who is HIV positive or bisexual or injects drugs; long-term residence or birth in an area with high prevalence of HIV infection; history of transfusion from 1978-1985; invasive cervical cancer; pregnancy. Offer to women seeking preconceptional care
• Influenza vaccine	Anyone who wishes to reduce the chance of becoming ill with influenza; resident in long-term care facility; chronic cardiopulmonary disorders; metabolic diseases (e.g., diabetes mellitus, hemoglobinopathies, immunosuppression, renal dysfunction); health-care workers; day-care workers; pregnant women who will be in the second or third trimester during the epidemic season. Pregnant women with medical problems should be offered vaccination before the influenza season regardless of stage of pregnancy
• Lipid profile assessment	Elevated cholesterol level; history of parent or sibling with blood cholesterol of at least 240 mg/dL; first degree relative with premature (<55 years of age for men, <65 years of age for women) coronary artery disease; diabetes mellitus; smoking habit

• Mammography	Women who have had breast cancer or who have a first-degree relative (ie, mother, sister, or daughter) or multiple other relatives who have a history of premenopausal breast or breast and ovarian cancer
• Measles, mumps, rubella vaccine	Adults born in 1957 or later should be offered vaccination (one dose of MMR) if there is no proof or immunity or documentation of a dose given after first birthday; persons vaccinated in 1963-1967 should be offered revaccination (2 doses); health-care workers, students entering college, international travelers, and rubella-negative postpartum patients should be offered a second dose
• Pneumococcal vaccine	Chronic illness such as cardiovascular disease, pulmonary disease, diabetes mellitus, alcoholism, chronic liver disease, cerebrospinal fluid leaks, functional or anatomic asplenia; exposure to an environment where pneumococcal outbreaks have occurred; immunocomprimised patients (eg, HIV infection, hematologic or solid malignancies, chemotherapy, steroid therapy); pregnant patients with chronic illness. Revaccination after 5 years may be appropriate for certain high-risk groups
• Rubella titer assessment	Childbearing age and no evidence of immunity
• STI testing	History of multiple sexual partners or a sexual partner with multiple contacts, sexual contact with persons with culture-proven STI, history of repeated episodes of STIs, attendance at clinics for STIs; routine screening for chlamydial and gonorrheal infection for all sexually active adolescents and other asymptomatic women at high risk for infection
• Skin examination	Increased recreational or occupational exposure to sunlight; family or personal history of skin cancer; clinical evidence of precursor lesions
• Thyroid-stimulating hormone test	Strong family history of thyroid disease; autoimmune disease (evidence of subclinical hypothyroidism may be related to unfavorable lipid profiles)
• Tuberculosis skin test	HIV infection; close contact with persons known or suspected to have TB; medical risk factors known to increase risk of disease if infected; born in country with high TB prevalence; medically underserved; low income; alcoholism; intravenous drug use; resident of long-term care facility (e.g., correctional institutions, mental institutions, nursing homes and facilities); health professional working in high-risk health-care facilities
• Varicella vaccine	All susceptible adults and adolescents, including health-care workers; household contacts of immunocompromised individuals; teachers; day-care workers; residents and staff of institutional settings, colleges, prisons, or military installations; international travellers; non-pregnant women of childbearing age

Advantages of counseling:

- Involves patient in his/her own care
- Dispels misconceptions, myths and rumors
- Improves success with complicated regimens
- Helps people change risky behaviors— a vital, yet difficult, task
- Facilitates the decision-making process regarding contraception and STI prevention
- Explains anticipated or possible side effects, which can help decrease anxiety and increase success with method
- Encourages clients to return if problems occur
- Reduces severity of serious complications through early recognition
- Builds and strengthens the provider/patient relationship

Principles of good counseling:

- *Listen*, look at your patients, repeat what you hear, and allow them to speak freely
- *Respect* and accept each individual
- *Allow plenty of time*
- Recognize the unique aspects of *each individual's situation*
- Ensure and maintain *confidentiality*
- Remain *sensitive* without becoming emotionally involved
- Be *nonjudgmental*
- Encourage *self-determination*
- Urge all your patients to *know* their HIV status
- Each encounter offers opportunity to counsel about STI/HIV prevention and contraception wherever encounter occurs. Particularly important during antepartum visits
- Inquire about problems patients may have had with previous medical recommendations; Learn from these experiences to improve success with your therapies
- Know what you are talking about! ◄──

The GATHER method suggests the following steps:

- **Greet** patient in a warm, friendly manner; help her to feel at ease
- **Ask** patient about her needs and reproductive goals; ask about risk for STIs
- **Tell** patient about her choices, explaining the advantages and disadvantages of all options
- **Help** patient to choose
- **Explain** the correct use of the method or drug being prescribed
- **Repeat** important instructions by the patient and clarify time and conditions of return visit

Reproductive/Contraceptive Goals:

GOAL:	MAIN CONTRACEPTIVE CONCERNS MAY BE:
Delaying birth of first child	Effectiveness of method, future fertility and STIs
Wants to avoid abortion for any reason	Need for maximal effectiveness; May want to use 2 methods consistently
Spacing births	Most convenient method; (Concern over failure of methods may be less)
Completed childbearing	Needs effective method for long term: offer IUD or sterilization as extremely effective methods

Taking Sexual Histories

Although historically health care providers have been reluctant to inquire about sexual issues because of both time and social constraints, more clinicians are realizing that sexual histories are essential to identifying at-risk individuals and to providing appropriate testing and treatment. Explain to the patient that obtaining sexual information is necessary to provide complete care, but reassure her that she has the right to discuss only what she is comfortable divulging. Patients often want correct sex information and need to discuss sexual concerns that may be affecting their sexual performance or satisfaction. Ask patients less direct questions in the beginning to build trust, then ask the questions that explicitly address sexual issues once you have their confidence. Answers may change as person becomes more comfortable. Ask those questions that will help you counsel or treat your patient. ◄

Initiating the Sexual History

- I will be asking some personal questions about your sexual activity to help me make more accurate diagnoses and to take better care of you
- Is this all right with you?
- You only need to tell me as much as you are comfortable sharing
- Your information is confidential
- Some patients have shared concerns with me related to their risks of infections or sexual activity. If you have any concerns, I would be happy to discuss them with you

Sexual History Questions

- **What are you doing to protect yourself from AIDS and other infections?** ◄
- Do you have questions regarding sex or sexual activity?
- How old were you when you had your first sexual experience?
- Are you sexually involved at this time?
- Do you have sex with men, women or both?
- Do you think you need contraception? How are you protecting yourself from pregnancy?
- How many sex partners have you had in the last 3 months? in the last 6 months? in your lifetime?
- How many sex partners does your partner have?
- Do you have penis in vagina sex, penis in mouth sex or penis in rectum sex?
- Do you drink alcohol or take drugs in association with sexual activity?
- Have you ever been forced or coerced to have sex?
- As a child, did anyone ever touch you genitals or ask you to touch theirs?
- Do you have sex for money, food, drugs or shelter?
- Do you enjoy sex? Do you have orgasms? Do you have pain with sex?
- Do you or your partner(s) have any sexual concerns?

Avoid Assumptions

Making assumptions about a patient's sexual behavior and orientation can leave out important information, undermine patient trust and make the patient feel judged or alienated, causing her to withhold information. This can result in diagnostic and treatment errors. Do not assume that patients:

- Are sexually active and need contraception
- Are NOT sexually active (e.g., older patients, young adolescents)
- Have current sexual partner(s)
- Are heterosexual, homosexual or bisexual
- Know if their partners have other partners
- Have the power to make contraceptive decisions ◄

FEMALE

Dyspareunia

- *Definition:* Pain during vaginal intercourse or vaginal penetration
- *Key questions:* Does she have pain with vaginal penetration? Does she have pain with early entry in the mid vaginal area? Is there pain with deep thrusting? Is pain occasional or consistent? With every partner? Does the pain change with different sexual positions? Is she aroused and lubricated before penetration?
- *Causes:* Organic - vestibulitis, urethritis/UTI, vaginitis, hypoestrogenism, PID, endometriosis, surgical scars or adhesions, pelvic injuries, tumors, hip joint or disc pain, female circumcision, orgasmic spasm
  Psychological - current or previous abuse, relationship stress, depression, anxiety, fear of sex
- *Treatment:* Directed to underlying pathology including depression. If dyspareunia is chronic, consider supplementing medical management with supportive counseling and sex therapy

Vaginismus (special case of dyspareunia)

- *Definition:* Painful involuntary spastic contraction of introital and pelvic floor muscles with attempted vaginal penetration
- *Causes:* Organic - may be secondary to current or previous dyspareunia and its causes. Psychological - sexual abuse, fears of abnormal anatomy (e.g. terror that vagina will rip with penile or speculum introduction), negative attitudes about sexuality
- *Treatment:* Education is critical. Insight into underlying causes helps. After source is recognized, start progressive desensitization exercises, which can include self manipulation and dilators. Sex therapist/psychologist intervention needed to deal with unconscious fears unresponsive to education

Decreased Libido (Hypoactive Sexual Desire)

- *Definition:* Relative lack of sexual desire defined by individual as troublesome to her sexual relationship; no absolute level "normal"
- *Causes:* Organic - may be due to acute or chronic debilitating medical condition (e.g., diabetes, stroke, spinal cord injury, arthritis, cancer, chronic obstructive pulmonary disease, coronary artery disease, etc.), medications (e.g. sedatives, narcotics, hypnotics, anticonvulsants, centrally-acting antihypertensives, tranquilizers, anorectics, and some antidepressants), dyspareunia, incontinence, alcohol, hormonal imbalance, or postpartum healing episiotomy
  Sexual practices - inadequate sexual stimulation or time for arousal. Sexual desires discordant with partner's desires (rule out hyperactive sexual desire disorder of partner). Psychological - depression, anxiety, exhaustion, life stress (finances, relationship problems, etc.), poor partner communications, lack of understanding about impacts of aging. Change in body image (breast-feeding, postpartum, weight gain, or post mastectomy or hysterectomy)
- *Treatment:* Treat underlying causes where possible. Rule out hyperactive sexual desire disorder of partner. Reassure about normalcy, if appropriate. Help patient create time and special space for sexual expression - no distractions from children, telephone, household chores. Suggest variety in sexual practices perhaps with aid of fantasies (romance novels are discreet source of fantasies for many women akin to Playboy for men). Physiologic androgen replacement can enhance libido. New drugs, including Viagra and ointments causing increased blood flow to the clitoris, are also under investigation. Consider referral to sex therapist

Excessive Sexual Desire (Hyperactive Sexual Desire)
- *Definition:* Excessive sexual activity resulting in social, psychological and physical problems. See Diagnostic and Statistical Manual of Mental Disorders, Fourth Edition (DSM-IV).
- *Cause:* Abuse at young age; attention seeking; acting out; other
- *Treatment:* Refer for psychological counseling and therapy

Orgasmic Disorders
- *Definitions:*
  - *Preorgasmia:* Never experienced orgasms and desires to be orgasmic
  - *Anorgasmia:* Orgasmic in past, no orgasms currently, desirous of orgasm
- *Cause:* Organic - may be secondary to dyspareunia, neurological, vascular disease, medications (e.g. sedatives, narcotics, hypnotics, anticonvulsants, centrally-acting antihypertensives, tranquilizers, anorectics, and some antidepressants - particularly SSRI class antidepressants), or poor sexual techniques of partner (painful, premature ejaculation) Psychological - negative attitude about sexuality, chronic relationship stress; lack of knowledge about body and sexual response
- *Treatment:* Treat underlying organic causes, if possible. Explain sexual response (suggest reading of ***Our Bodies Ourselves***). Add behavioral/psychological approach using PLISST model (see vi), and sensate focusing exercises. Help couple set alternative pleasuring goals. Refer to sex therapist if initial interventions not successful

MALE

Decreased Libido (Hypoactive sexual desire disorder)
- No absolute level "normal"; "decreased libido" usually related to previous experience
- Evaluation and treatment similar to female's (see above).

Premature Ejaculation
- *Definition:* Persistent or recurrent ejaculation before, upon or shortly after vaginal penetration. Ejaculation occurs earlier than patient or partner desires. Average time from intromission to ejaculation in "normal" couples is 2 minutes; shorter interval is consistent with diagnosis.
- *Causes:* Organic - urethritis, prostatitis, neurological disease (e.g. multiple sclerosis). Psychological - learned behavior, result of anxiety (especially among teens).
- *Treatment:* Education and reassurance is important. If goal is pleasuring of partner, teach other techniques to arouse her prior to intercourse. "Start and stop" technique can be used to prolong erection; man stops stimulation for at least 30 seconds when he feels ejaculation imminent. "Squeeze" technique helpful; when man feels impending ejaculation, partner firmly squeezes the head of the penis beneath the glans for 4-5 seconds to decrease erection. Selective serotonin reuptake inhibitors (SSRIs) in low doses may be helpful if these other techniques are not adequate. Refer to sex therapist (or urologist if cause organic) for additional treatment if needed

Delayed (Retarded) Ejaculation
- *Definition:* Inability to or difficulty in experiencing orgasm and ejaculation with a partner
- *Cause:* usually psychological; learned behavior; may occur when a man has masturbatory patterns that cannot be duplicated with partner; overemphasis on sexual performance. Rule out organic problems carefully.
- *Treatment:* referral to sex therapist recommended

Erectile Dysfunction/Disorders (ED) (Impotence)
- *Definition:* Inability to attain or sustain an erection that is satisfactory for coitus
- *Primary:* never achieved erection
  - *Causes:* Organic - low testosterone levels due to hypothalamic-pituitary-testicular disorder; severe vascular compromise. Psychological - usual cause
- *Secondary:* inability to currently attain erection (may be situational)
  - *Causes:* Organic - diabetes mellitus, alcohol abuse, hypothyroidism, drug dependency, medications (e.g. sedatives, narcotics, hypnotics, anticonvulsants, centrally-acting antihypertensives, tranquilizers, anorectics, and some antidepressants), hypopituitarism, penile infections, atherosclerosis, aortic aneurysm, muscular sclerosis, spinal cord lesions, orchiectomy or prostatectomy

  Psychological - depression, relationship stress, prior abuse, etc. Suspect when patient has morning erection or is able to masturbate to ejaculation
- *Treatment:* Treat underlying cause. Switch medications if possible. Same measures which help women's sexual desire may be useful to try. Medical or mechanical treatments available:
  1. *Testosterone.* Shown to be useful in wasting diseases (AIDS) and other low testosterone conditions. Available in patches for ease of use
  2. *Sildenafil citrate (Viagra)* 25-100 mg (usual dose 50 mg) tablet one hour prior to intercourse. Contraindicated with other ED treatments, retinosis pigmentosa, priapism or nitrates (nitroglycerin, isosorbide mononitrate, isosorbide nitrate, pentaerythritol tetranitrate, erythrityl tetranitrate)
  3. *Alprostadil injections (Edex or Caverject)* prostaglandin E1 ~ 1 cc injected into corpus cavernosa (strengths 125 µg - 1000 µg. Dose determined in office visit.) Excessive injection may cause priapism. Erection achieved with stimulation lasts 30-60 minutes. Avoid in anticoagulated patients and with vasoactive medications. Limit 3 per week
  4. *Alprostadil suppository (Muse)* prostaglandin pellet E1 (125-1000 µg) placed inside urethra. Erection occurs as drug absorbed. 70% successful. Contraindications - anatomical penile abnormalities (strictures, hypospadias, etc.), and thrombosis risk factors. Limit 2/day
  5. *Yohimbine hydrochloride.* Prescription pill composed of indole alkaloid. Modestly successful. Avoid in psychiatric patients (causes agitation and hallucination).
  6. *Vacuum Erection Device (VED).* Use of a vacuum pump and different size rubber bands maintains an erection for 30 minutes. Safe and effective (90% success rate). May be cumbersome and decrease spontaneity
  7. *Penile implants (prostheses).* Bendable rods or inflatable reservoirs permanently implanted surgically into penis. Activated/inflated for intercourse. Success rate high, but associated with surgical risks and the risk that natural erections disappear
  8. *Microsurgery.* Used in men with atherosclerosis of penile arteries or venous pathology; over 50% success rate

Adolescents are very interested in sex, contraception, and STIs, but they rarely raise these issues with their providers. Although sexual abstinence is increasing among teens, most American adolescents have had intercourse before high school graduation. Helping adolescents to grow in self respect, positive self-image is the most important goal of all work with teens.

COUNSELING CHALLENGES POSED BY ADOLESCENTS

Teens are not "young adults". Developmentally appropriate approaches are needed
- Age 12-14 – teens are very concrete, egocentric (self-focused) and concerned with personal appearance and acceptance and have a short attention span
- Age 14-15 – teens are peer oriented and authority resistant (challenge boundaries) and have very limited images of the future
- Age 16-17 – teens are developing logical thought processes and goals for the future

Nonjudgmental, open-ended and reflective questions are better than direct yes-no inquiries. Try reflective questions such as "What would you want to tell a friend who was thinking about having sex?" instead of "You're not having sex, are you?".

CONFIDENTIALITY

Adolescents are often afraid to obtain medical care for contraception, pregnancy testing or STI treatment because they fear parental reaction. Over two-thirds of teens never discuss anything sexual that they have done with their parents; over one-half felt their parents could not handle it. All teens should be entitled to confidential services and counseling but billing systems and/or laws in some states affect their confidential access to family planning services. Know your local laws and refer to sites that may be able to meet all the teen's needs if your practice can not.

ADOLESCENTS AND THE LAW

This table provides information on an adolescent's right to consent to reproductive health, contraception, and abortion services.

Table 6.1 Adolescents and the Law

AL ●○■	DC ●	IA ●○★	MI ●■	NH ●○	OK ●	TX ●○★
AK ●□	FL ☆	KS ●○★	MN ●★	NJ ●○☆	OR ●	UT ●○★
AZ ●	GA ●★	KY ●■	MS ●■	NM ●○	PA ●○■	VT ●
AR ●○★	HI ●	LA ●■	MO ●○■	NY ●○	RI ●○■	VA ●★
CA ●○	ID ●■	ME ●	MT ○☆	NC ●■	SC ●■	WA ●○
CO ●☆	IL ☆	MD ●★	NE ●○★	ND ●○■	SD ●○★	WV ●★
CT ●○	IN ●○■	MA ●○■	NV ○☆	OH ●○★	TN ●■	WI ●■
DE ●★						WY ●■

● = Minor explicitly authorized to consent to contraceptive and/or STD/HIV services

○ = No law or policy exists for minor consent to contraceptive services

■ = Parental consent required for minors seeking abortion (a parent or legal guardian must be present during the abortion)

□ = Parental consent requirements are enjoined (prohibited or declared unenforceable by courts)

★ = Parental notification required for minors seeking abortion (parent or legal guardian must sign a statement stating the parent has been notified that an abortion is to be performed on the minor)

☆ = Parental notification requirements are enjoined (prohibited or declared unenforceable by courts)

Sources: *The Status of Major Abortion-Related Laws and Policies in the States, October 2000*, Alan Guttmacher Institute. *Issues In Brief: Minors and the Right to Consent to Health Care*, Alan Guttmacher Institute, 2000.

Note: In all but four states, the age of majority is 18. In Alabama and Nevada, it is 19, and in Pennsylvania and Missouri, it is 21; however, in Missouri 18 is the age of consent for health care. Many of the laws contain specific clauses that affect their meaning and application. The authors encourage readers to consult the above documents for more details (see www.agi-usa.org).

ADOLESCENTS AS RISK TAKERS

- Full evaluation of behaviors is important to personalize counseling. Teens must move away from parental authority figures to become independent adult individuals, but, along the way, they may take excessive risks
- HEADSS interview technique helpful as an organized approach. Ask each teen about Home, Education, Activities, Drugs, Sexuality (activity, orientation and abuse) and Suicide
- Guidelines for Adolescent Preventive Services (GAPS) developed to help health care providers encourage adolescents to prevent or modify health-compromising behaviors.
- Look for the triad: eating disorders, amenorrhea and osteoporosis

SEX EDUCATION

The sex education, contraception and STIs curricula offered in many schools are frequently not medically correct, and many students have only superficial understanding of what these topics mean to them. Information teens obtain from peers is also often inaccurate, and myths abound:

- *You cannot get pregnant the first time you have intercourse*
- *You cannot get pregnant if you douche after sex*
- *Having a baby makes you a woman, makes your boyfriend love you, and gets you the attention you deserve. Your baby will love you*
- *Making a girl pregnant means that you are a man*

Adolescents need very concrete information and opportunities to role play and practice:

- How to open and place a condom and where to carry it
- How to negotiate NOT having sex ←
- How to negotiate condom use with sex partner
- How to punch out the pills and where to keep the pack
- How to move in direction of dual protection: condoms and another contraceptive ←
- How to remember when to return for Depo-Provera
- How to use emergency contraception

ADOLESCENT HEALTH RESOURCES
American Medical Association: (800) 621-8335

AMA Guidelines for Adolescent Preventive Services (GAPS): Recommendations and Rationale
- Provides review of the scientific basis for recommendations

GAPS Clinical Evaluation and Management Handbook.
- Presents an algorithmic approach to diagnosis and management of GAPS conditions

DAPS Implementation and Resource Manual.
- Identifies resources for health guidance materials, confidentiality, and practical strategies for implementation

GAPS Implementation Forms.
- Reproducible forms, including adolescent and parent questionnaires, preventive services tracking chart, body mass index charts, blood pressure graphs, and health guidance prompt sheets

Internet
- Adolescent Health On-Line: www.ama-assn.org/adolhlth/adolhlth.htm
- Division of Adolescent and School Health, National Center for Chronic Disease Prevention and Health Promotion, Centers for Disease Control and Prevention: www.cdc.gov/nccdphp/dash/index.htm
- Society for Adolescent Medicine: www.adolescenthealth.org

PERIMENOPAUSE

The period of time (average 46-51 years of age) toward the end of the reproductive life of a woman when her ovarian follicles are less responsive to stimulation. The single marker of the perimenopause is menstrual irregularity. Fluctuations in ovarian hormonal production can result in intermittent vasomotor symptoms, menstrual disturbances and reduced fertility. It is important to remember, though, that even with reduced fertility, a perimenopausal woman needs contraception until she is truly menopause. Perimenopausal women have the highest abortion rate (# abortions/# pregnancies) of any age group except women under 15

- All methods of birth control are available to eligible women until menopause.
- Sterilization is popular in the group. 50% of all contracepting women age 40-44 have been sterilized and another 20% have a partner with a vasectomy
- Oral contraceptive pills or combined injections (Lunelle) will provide hot flash relief and cycle control for eligible women. Smokers may use DMPA with ERT add-back. Estrogen-containing contraceptives should not be used in women over 35 who smoke

Health Screening: see Chapter 2 for screening guidelines by age

MENOPAUSE

The permanent cessation of spontaneous menses. Average age 51-52. Menopause creates an excellent opportunity to encourage healthy diets, exercise and health-promoting lifestyles (smoking cessation, calcium supplementation, etc.) Perhaps the single most important lifestyle message is that women who smoke as little as 1-4 cigarettes/day have a 2.5 fold increased risk of fatal coronary artery disease *[Speroff - 1999, p. 649]*

Common Physiologic Changes After Estrogen Loss

- Hot flashes
- Sleep disturbances
- Mood swings, decreased ability to concentrate and remember
- Thinning of genital urinary tissue (atrophic vaginitis, urinary incontinence)
- Osteopenia, osteoporosis, increased risk for fracture
- Increased risk for cardiovascular disease, unfavorable lipid profiles, increased vascular resistance, increased homocysteine levels
- Other possible consequences of estrogen deficiency: increased risk of Alzheimer's disease, colon cancer, tooth loss, macular degenerative eye disease

HORMONE REPLACEMENT THERAPY (HRT)

Each women should be informed of potential benefits and risks of hormone replacement therapy individualized to her own situation as part of a comprehensive health promotion program which also emphasizes proper nutrition and exercise. HRT is therapeutic in relieving vaso-motor symptoms but is also used as preventive therapy to reduce the long term sequelae of estrogen deficiency: increased risk of vertebral, radial and femoral head fracture, and genital atrophy. 60% of females between the ages of 55-64 are sexually active. HRT (estrogen) helps alleviate decreased lubrication and genital atrophy. Use of HRT in recently menopausal women *may* prevent later decline in cognitive function.

PRESCRIBING PRECAUTIONS

- Pregnancy
- Undiagnosed abnormal vaginal bleeding
- Active liver disease or chronic impaired liver function
- Recent or active thrombophlebitis or thromboembolic disorders (unless anticoagulated)
- Breast cancer or known or suspected estrogen-dependent neoplasm

• Recent myocardial infarction or severe cardiac artery disease

STARTING HRT

- Patient counseling is key to success with HRT. Clearly describe onset of action of HRT for women with hot flashes as well as side effects (especially vaginal spotting and bleeding)
- Answer all questions about possible risks (especially her concerns about breast cancer)
- Recent routine history and physical examination sufficient to identify any contraindications.
- Usual well-woman care measures (e.g. mammogram, pap smear, lipid profile) should be provided but are not essential prior to starting HRT. Endometrial biopsy not needed except when evaluating abnormal vaginal bleeding
- Women <1-2 years since LMP who plan to use combined continuous HRT can use progestin withdrawal (MPA 5-10 mg per day for 14 days) prior to HRT start to slough existing endometrium
- Older women who have not had estrogen for years appreciate a slow start—easing over time into physiologic replacement doses to reduce side effects
- Women who have had oophorectomy may need androgen supplementation
- Selection of a hormone replacement preparation depends on the patient's therapeutic goals, personal preferences and potential side effects. The greatest clinical experience about long term health benefits has come from the use of conjugated equine estrogens. The increasing numbers of HRT products allows greater flexibility in individualizing therapy to meet each patient's needs

Generic names - Estrogens	Brand names
Conjugated estrogen tablets, USP	Premarin®
Synthetic conjugated estrogens, A tablets	Cenestin®
Esterified estrogens tablets	Estratab®, Menest®
Estropipate tablets	Ogen®, Ortho-est®
Estradiol tablets	Estrace®
Matrix estradiol transdermal systems	Alora®, Climara®, FemPatch®, Vivelle™, Esclim
Reservoir estradiol transdermal systems	Estraderm®

Generic names - Progestins	Brand names
Medroxyprogesterone acetate (MPA) tablets	Amen®, Curretab®, Cycrin®, Provera®
Megestrol acetate tablets	Megace®
Norethindrone tablets	Micronor®, Nor-QD®, Norlutin®
Norethindrone acetate tablets	Aygestin®
Micronized progesterone capsules	Prometrium®
Progesterone vaginal gel	Crinone®

Generic names - Combined Products	Brand names
17 β estradiol and micronized norgestimate tablets	Ortho-Prefest®
Conjugated estrogens and MPA tablets	Premphase®, Prempro®
Esterified estrogens and methyl testosterone tablets	Estratest®, Estratest® H.S.
Ethinyl estradiol and norethindrone acetate tablets	Femhrt®
Estradiol and norethindrone acetate tablets	Activella™
Matrix estradiol/ norethindrone acetate transdermal systems	CombiPatch™

FOLLOW-UP

- Patient should return in 1-3 months to answer further questions/manage side effects
- Have the woman keep a menstrual calendar of any breakthrough bleeding or spotting
- If reductions are needed in estrogen dosing, move slowly.
- Be available to answer questions when the media publish alarms about HRT safety and whenever she has questions
- Routine well-woman care is sufficient. No special monitoring measures are needed

Ideally, planning should involve both a woman and her partner ←
Long before pregnancy, women should start taking folic acid ←

Assess:
- Reproductive, family and personal medical and surgical history with attention to pelvic surgeries
- Smoking, drug use, alcohol use: advise to stop and refer to help if needed
- Nutrition habits: identify excesses or inadequacies
- Medications: make adjustments in those that may affect fertility and/or pregnancy outcome. Advise patient not to make any changes without clinician's knowledge
- Age, risk for sexually transmitted infection/infertility
- Impacts of any medications (over-the-counter, prescription, herbal). Use of Acutane ← for acne requires extremely effective contraception and strong consideration of the use of 2 contraceptives correctly and consistently

Offer Screening for:
- Infections (TB, gonorrhea, chlamydia, HIV, syphilis, Hepatitis B & C, as per CDC guidelines). Consider vaginal wet mount if discharge present
- Neoplasms (breast, cervical dysplasia, warts, etc.)
- Immunity (rubella, tetanus, chicken pox, HBV)

Provide Genetic Counseling:
- Advanced maternal age
- Sickle cell anemia, thalassemia
- Tay-Sachs, Canavan disease
- Previous poor pregnancy outcomes
- Family history of mental retardation or genetic disorders
- Alcohol use, tobacco use, substance abuse
- Cystic fibrosis
- Seizure disorders
- Diabetes, neural tube defects
- Other heritable medical problems

Assess Environmental Hazards:
- Chemical, radioactive and infectious exposures at workplace, home, hobbies
- Physical conditions, especially workplace

Assess Psychosocial Factors:
- Readiness of woman and partner for parenthood
- Mental health (depression, etc.) and domestic violence
- Financial issues and support systems

Recommend:

- Balanced diet
- Prenatal vitamin with 0.4 mg folic acid for all women (use higher dose folic acid, 1-4 mg, in higher-risk women such as women with previous neural tube defect, diet with minimal vegetable intake, alcoholic, malabsorption or on anticonvulsants)
- Minimize STI exposure risk
- Weight loss, if obese (gradual loss until conception)
- Moderate exercise

Avoid

- Raw meat (including fish) and unpasteurized dairy products
- Abdominal/pelvic X-rays, if possible
- Excesses in diet, vitamins, exercise
- Unusual foods (pica), herbs, etc.
- Sex with multiple partners or sex with a partner who may be HIV-positive or ⬅ have other STI. Use condom if any question

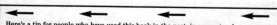

Here's a tip for people who have used this book in the past: in one or two hours you can find the major changes in this text. Simply thumb through the pages looking for the arrows! This would also be an excellent way to give a lecture on "what's new in family planning."

Early testing gives a woman a head start to pursue pregnancy options
- Prenatal care can be initiated promptly
- Ectopic pregnancies may be detected earlier
- Full menu of elective options available

PREGNANCY TESTS*

Urine tests:
- *Enzyme-linked immunosorbent assay (ELISA) test:*
  - Immunometric test uses antibody specific to β subunit of placentally-produced HCG and another antibody to produce a color change. Commonly used in home pregnancy test and in offices and clinics
  - Performed in 1-3 minutes using urine samples
  - Test turns positive at levels of 25 mIU/ml. This level can be detectable 7-10 days after conception, which is 1-2 days after implantation in some pregnancies. May require 5-7 days after implantation to detect all pregnancies

Serum tests (blood drawn):
- *Radioimmunoassay:*
  - Uses radioisotopes, which detect β-HCG levels as low as 5 mIU/ml
  - Results available in 1-2 hours
  - Offers ability to quantify levels of β-HCG to monitor levels over time when clinically indicated
* See p. 642 of *Contraceptive Technology (17th edition)* for a chart on all clinical pregnancy tests

HCG QUICK FACTS

- β-HCG can be detected as early as 7-10 days after conception but pregnancy cannot be ruled out until 7 days after expected menses
- A sensitive (urine or serum) pregnancy test can be positive 1-2 days after implantation
- In a normal pregnancy, β-HCG values double every 1.5 days before 5 weeks gestation and every 2 days between 5-7 weeks.
- If needed for evaluation of early pregnancy, serial β-HCG testing should be done every 1-2 days until levels reach discriminatory levels of 1800-2000 MIu/ml, when a gestational sac can be visualized reliably by vaginal ultrasound
- Average time for β-HCG levels to become non-detectable after first trimester abortion (medical or surgical) ranges from 31-38 days

MANAGEMENT TIPS

- Home tests can be misused or misinterpreted. Don't make clinical decisions based on home test results
- ELISA tests can have false-negative results at low levels. If in doubt, repeat urine test in 1-2 days or obtain serum tests with a quantitative β-HCG radioimmunoassay

PREGNANCY TEST NEGATIVE: A TEACHABLE MOMENT

A negative pregnancy test for a woman *not* wanting to become pregnant clearly provides the counselor or clinician with a teachable moment.

"Phew! The pregnancy test is negative." This must have been scary to worry that you might be pregnant.

1. If you haven't been using contraception, this is your "wake-up call." What would work best for you in the future?
2. Abstinence may be your chosen path now; if not, use contraception unless you want to become pregnant.
3. Learn about emergency contraceptive pills and emergency IUD insertion
4. Don't even think of trying to become pregnant in order to see if you can become pregnant.
5. Take the path less traveled sexually from this moment on: never, just never, have intercourse without knowing that you are protected against both infection and unintended or unwanted pregnancy.
6. Remember, your negative urine pregnancy test is not accurate for acts of intercourse in the past 2 weeks.

PREGNANCY TEST POSITIVE: A TEACHABLE MOMENT

The pregnancy test is positive and she wants to continue the pregnancy. Whether or not this pregnancy was planned*, your patient's mind is made up: she will continue this pregnancy, providing you, the counselor or clinician, with a teachable moment.

The pregnancy test is positive and she will continue her pregnancy to term

1. Start folic acid (0.4 mg) in prenatal vitamins today. Buy some prenatal vitamins on the way home.
2. Stop drinking alcohol today.
3. Stop smoking today.
4. Find the person who will follow you during your pregnancy and tell your health care provider if you are on any medication.
5. Use condoms if at any risk for HIV or other STIs.
6. Eat well. Gain 25-30 pounds during your pregnancy.

* If she doesn't want to continue pregnancy, discuss pregnancy termination options or refer her to someone else who would feel comfortable doing this.

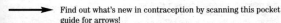

Find out what's new in contraception by scanning this pocket guide for arrows!

CHAPTER 10

Postpartum Contraception

www.avsc.org or www.fhi.org ◄—

Because ovulation may return within 3-6 weeks postpartum (before a woman realizes she is at risk), planning for postpartum contraception should begin during pregnancy and use should be initiated as early as possible postpartum. A newborn can place many demands on a woman's time, so her method should be as convenient for her to use as possible. Some postpartum women will choose to return to the use of abstinence as their contraceptive. Some women don't have ◄— the "choice" to be abstinent or are afraid their partners will go elsewhere if they don't have sex.

AT DELIVERY

- Tubal sterilization may be performed (at C-section or after vaginal delivery)
- IUD may be inserted within 20 minutes of delivery of placenta (requires special equipment/training)

PRIOR TO LEAVING HOSPITAL

- Breast-feeding should be encouraged. Reinforce education about lactational amenorrhea if patient interested (see Chapter 15, p. 40-43)
- Pelvic rest (no douching, no sex, no tampons) is generally recommended for 4-6 weeks. Many women choose NOT to follow this advice in spite of increased risk for infection. Some clinicians encourage women to become sexually active when they feel comfortable and ready
- Women are strongly advised to abstain from intercourse until lochia stopped
  Contraception should be provided in advance of a woman's need postpartum with any of the following:
    - Tubal sterilization
    - Progestin-only methods: Norplant, Depo-Provera, progestin-only (mini) pills
    - **NOTE:** These methods may prolong postpartum bleeding. Women who have low hemoglobin values may benefit from a 2-week delay in initiation of progestin-only methods. Women with history of or high risk for postpartum depression may benefit from similar delays. See page 35 for discussion of other hypothetical concerns for breastfeeding women
    - Male or female condoms or spermicides (to reduce risk of pelvic infection)
    - Withdrawal
    - COCs and Lunelle may be prescribed for nonlactating women starting 3-4 weeks postpartum (risk of thrombosis associated with pregnancy reduced by that time)
    - Emergency contraceptive pills may be provided in advance

AT POSTPARTUM VISIT (3-6 WEEKS)

- Encourage breast feeding
- Lactational amenorrhea follow-up. Provide condoms as transitional method PRN return of menses, decrease in breast-feeding, etc
- Emergency contraception may be given if needed
- Progestin-only methods may be provided (Norplant, Depo-Provera, progestin-only pills). Provide back-up method as needed if initiated when not on menses
- Combined oral contraceptive pills or combined injectables may be started unless woman is exclusively breast-feeding. Provide backup method as needed
- IUD may be inserted if uterus well involuted (whether or not she is breast-feeding)
- Condoms (male or female) may be given as primary or backup contraceptive to provide STI risk reduction; withdrawal can be used at any time
- Tubal ligation may be provided after uterine involution
- Diaphragm/cervical cap may be fitted after pelvis/cervix return to normal configuration
- NFP and FAM should await resumption of normal cycles

OVERVIEW

The availability of safe elective abortion procedures is important for fertility control; 48% of pregnancies in this country are unintended. The same methods can be applied to pregnancies that need to be terminated for medical reasons.

Despite having one of the highest abortion rates among developed countries, in 1995, over 78% of US counties had no abortion providers or facilities. Many state laws impose mandatory restrictions, waiting periods, and consent requirements. For current information on your state's abortion laws, contact National Abortion Rights Action League (NARAL) (202-973-3000 or www.naral.org/) for a copy of "A State-By-State Review of Abortion and Reproductive Rights". Approximately 1.2 million abortions are performed in the U.S. each year; 88% are first trimester and 97% are surgical.

Surgical abortion techniques (especially vacuum aspiration) have a proven safety profile, with serious morbidity in less than 1% of procedures and a death rate of 0.5/100,000 women (compared to maternal mortality with a continued pregnancy of approximately 8/100,000 women). The introduction of several agents for early medical abortion have added new options. In the US, methotrexate and misoprostol are currently available; mifepristone - RU-486 (a progesterone antagonist) was approved in October 2000.

Second trimester abortions are not discussed in this chapter. For more information see *Contraceptive Technology*

Features of Medical and Surgical Abortion

Medical	Surgical
Generally avoids invasive procedure	Involves invasive procedure
Requires multiple visits	Usually requires one visit
Days to weeks to complete	Usually complete in a predictable period of time
Available during early pregnancy	Available during early and later pregnancy
High success rate (95%)	High success rate (98% - 99%)
Requires follow-up to ensure completion of abortion	Does not require follow-up in all cases
May be more private in some circumstances; will vary for each individual patient	May be more private in some circumstances; will vary for each individual patient
Patient participation in multi-step process	Less patient participation in a single-step process
	Allows use of sedation, if desired

ELECTIVE SURGICAL ABORTION

DESCRIPTION

Voluntary termination of pregnancy using vacuum aspiration in early gestations. In later gestations (after 14 weeks) with instrumented tissue removal (forceps).

EFFECTIVENESS

- 98-99% effective; failures are mostly incomplete abortions with small amounts of retained tissue; rarely does the pregnancy continue

PROCEDURE

- After informed consent obtained according to local law, type of procedure is determined by gestational age
- May dilate the cervix with an osmotic mechanical dilator such as laminaria if > 12 weeks ◀
  or with a prostaglandin such as misoprostol with or without laminaria in second trimester
- Antibiotic prophylaxis may significantly reduce risk of post-procedure infection. Doxycycline 200 mg 30-60 minutes prior to procedure and 100 mg orally twice a day for 3 days, or metronidazole 1 g preoperatively and 500 mg orally every 6 hours for 3 doses. Recent study in Los Angeles showed nearly 1 in 5 women seeking pregnancy termination had chlamydial cervicitis; bacterial vaginosis rates are high also. In areas of high chlamydia prevalence, a 7-day course of doxycycline, or a single dose of azithromycin 1 g may be given preoperatively
- Cleanse ectocervix and endocervix
- Administer cervical anesthesia; if desired, adjunctive conscious sedation can also be used. Adding a small dose of vasopressin (5 units) to cervical anesthetic significantly reduces risk of hematometra
- Place tenaculum and mechanically dilate cervix if not previously dilated
- Using sterile technique, insert a plastic tube to fundus and apply suction to aspirate products of conception
- May confirm adequacy of procedure by checking for rasp with a sharp curette (optional)
- Evaluate tissue to confirm presence of placental villi/gestational sac if early pregnancy. If more than 9 weeks should be able to visualize fetal tissue
- Administer Rh immune globulin if woman is Rh negative

COST

	Managed-Care Setting	Public Provider Setting
<12 weeks	unknown	$130 - 800 ◀
12-26 weeks	unknown	$400 - 2000 ◀

The equipment for MVA (manual vacuum aspiration surgical abortion) is quite inexpensive, easily portable and could lower the cost of surgical abortion significantly.

ADVANTAGES

- Provides woman with reproductive choice
- Ability to prevent an unwanted or defective birth or a halt pregnancy that poses risk to maternal health
- Safe and rapid; preoperative evaluation and procedure can usually be done in a single visit from a medical perspective (local legal restrictions may affect this)
- No increase in risk of breast cancer, infertility, cervical incompetence, preterm labor, or congenital anomalies in subsequent pregnancy after uncomplicated first-trimester abortion
- Safer for maternal health than continuing pregnancy
- Can be provided as early as intrauterine pregnancy is diagnosed

DISADVANTAGES

- Most women experience cramping and pain with procedure; the noise of the vacuum machine may cause significant anxiety
- Possibility of later regret (also is true for undesired pregnancy that is continued; good pre-procedure counseling can reduce)
- See complications

COMPLICATIONS

- Infection <1%
- Incomplete abortion 0.5%-1.0%; Failed abortion 0.1%-0.5%
- Hemorrhage 0.03%-1.0%
- Post-abortal syndrome (hematometra) <1%
- Asherman's syndrome rare (usually in setting of septic abortion)
- Infertility an uncommon complication, related to PID or Asherman's syndrome
- Mortality: Elective abortion <1 per 100,000 (vs. Pregnancy/childbirth 8/100,000)

CANDIDATES FOR USE

- Any woman requesting abortion. State laws often limit gestational age (typically less than 24 weeks) ◄
- *Adolescents:* State laws vary regarding requirements and consent requirements (See p. 16)

INITIATING METHOD

- Carefully discuss all pregnancy options, including prenatal care for parenting or for adoption and programs available for assistance with each option
- If patient chooses abortion, discuss available techniques when applicable (surgical versus medical)
- Obtain informed consent after answering all questions
- Offer emotional support, education, pre- and post-procedural instructions, and contraception
- Usually perform procedure in outpatient setting unless woman has severe medical problems requiring more intense monitoring or deeper anesthesia

INSTRUCTIONS FOR PATIENT

- Keep telephone number(s) nearby for any emergencies
- May resume usual activities same day if procedure done under local anesthesia
- One week pelvic rest (no tampons, douching or sexual intercourse)
- Use NSAIDs or acetaminophen for cramping, NSAIDs or ergotamine (methergine) for bleeding
- Showers, baths and swimming are permitted
- Seek medical care urgently if heavy bleeding, excessive cramping, fevers, chills, or malodorous discharge
- Use contraception if sexually active and keep EC available for future use

FOLLOW-UP

_Have you had a temperature >100.4°F
_What has your bleeding been like since the procedure?
_Have you had any new abdominal or pelvic pain?

PROBLEM MANAGEMENT
Infection
- Patients who develop endometritis can generally be treated using outpatient PID therapies described in the CDC Guidelines (see Chapter 35 p. 139).
- Cases that are more complicated may require hospitalization and intravenous antibiotics.
- Always evaluate possibility of retained products and need for reaspiration

Persistent or excessive bleeding
- *Uterine atony* - Rule out retained products and infection. Use uterine-contracting agents (prostaglandin analogues) or vascular constricting agents (methergine)
- *Cervical laceration* - Suture external tears if bleeding significantly, tamponade endocervical lacerations with inflated Foley balloon or similar device or clamp area
- *Retained products of conception* - Gentle reaspiration. Provide antibiotics
- *Uterine perforation* - Observe closely; evaluate surgically if any concern about bowel perforation or vascular injury; give antibiotics ⟵
- *Hemorrhage* - transfuse to replace large blood loss; provide blood factors to patients with coagulopathies. In rare cases, may need to provide uterine tamponade while transporting to center for treatment (e.g. embolization, hysterectomy, etc.)

Post-abortal syndrome
- Hematometra (intrauterine clots after procedure). Painful. Blood may not be visible vaginally. Most common at 9-11 weeks. Treat with repeat suction curettage and methyl ergonovine maleate for 1-3 days. Adding small doses of vasopressin to cervical anesthesia at time of initial procedure reduces risk

Failed abortion
- Can be due to uterine anomaly or ectopic pregnancy. Obtain ultrasound. Repeat procedure if indicated

Incomplete abortion/retained products of conception
- Reaspirate

FERTILITY AFTER USE
- Immediate return to baseline fertility. Contraceptive should be supplied immediately

ELECTIVE MEDICAL ABORTION WITH METHOTREXATE & MISOPROSTOL

DESCRIPTION
Combination medical agents:
- Methotrexate (MTX) is administered first to prevent continued implantation of the pregnancy. Dose: 50 mg/m² OR empirically 50 mg.
- Misoprostol (MIS) is given 3-7 days later to induce expulsion of the products of conception.

EFFECTIVENESS
- Complete abortion rate 95% up to 49 days gestation (rates drop to 84% if 50-56 days)
- Like surgical abortion, most failures are incomplete abortions; continuing pregnancy is rare
- 12-35% of women have 20-30 day delay in abortion

MECHANISMS
- MTX prevents reduction of folic acid to tetrahydrofolate by binding to dihydrofolate reductase. This prevents proliferation of placental villi by interfering with DNA synthesis.
- The addition of MIS increases uterine contractions to expel the products of conception

COST

Drug costs: Parenteral MTX + intravaginal MIS $10-12

                  Oral MTX + intravaginal MIS $23

- Also add cost of office visits (with ultrasound) and follow-up needed if unsuccessful

ADVANTAGES

- Provides a woman with reproductive choice (see ELECTIVE SURGICAL ABORTION, p. 26-28)
- Very early abortions can be performed
- Potentially private method
- Therapeutic for ectopic pregnancy in 90-95% of cases
- Less risk of operative complications (risk present only if aspiration required)
- Some women feel more in control of procedure, feel it is more "natural"
- Provides option to women who may not have surgical options (although need to have provider available to perform suction curretage if required)
- Very well liked by women who desire this alternative to surgical abortion

DISADVANTAGES

- Cramping, abdominal pain, nausea (3-66%), vomiting (2-25%), diarrhea (3-52%), fever and chills (8-60%). 40-90% of women take pain reliever
- Vaginal bleeding averages 10-17 days
- May be up to 1 month delay before abortion is complete
- Methotrexate (MTX) and misoprostol (MIS) are Class X drugs (teratogens); follow-up is mandatory to ensure that the abortion is complete
- See COMPLICATIONS

COMPLICATIONS

- Failed abortion (continuing pregnancy with exposure to Class X teratogen)
- Incomplete abortion
- Approximately 5% will require surgical abortion
- Hemorrhage (women may experience blood clots as may some women during a normal menstrual period)
- Infection
- Neutropenia, stomatitis or oral ulcers (< 1%) ◄━━━

CANDIDATES FOR USE

- Pregnant women, gestational age ≤ 49 days (well dated by LMP and/or ultrasound) desiring medical termination of pregnancy
- Women willing to abstain from sexual intercourse, alcohol and folate supplements for two weeks and to comply with visit schedule
- Women who are not anemic

INITIATING METHOD

- Carefully discuss all pregnancy options, including prenatal care for parenting or for adoption and highlight programs available for assistance with each option
- If patient chooses elective abortion, discuss available techniques (surgical vs. medical)
- Review protocol, risks, benefits and visit schedule
- Assess patient's access to provider if D&C is needed
- Obtain informed consent after all questions are answered

Protocol (adapted from National Abortion Federation Guidelines):

Day 1: Baseline labs including blood type with Rh, hemoglobin (liver function tests and creatinine, if clinically indicated); gestational age ≤ 49 days. Vaginal ultrasound to confirm dates if available. Administer MTX 50 mg/m² body surface area IM or 50 mg orally

Day 3-7: MIS 800 µg. Patient self-inserts tablets into posterior fornix of vagina (usually 4 x 200 mg tabs - some clinicians have found they are more effective when each tablet is broken in half). Administer Rh immunoglobulin, if Rh negative

Day 8: Ultrasound; if sac present, repeat dose of MIS (800 mg)

Day 15: Follow-up; repeat ultrasound if abortion not confirmed at prior visit:
- If gestational cardiac activity present, perform D&C
- If only sac present, return in 3 weeks (day 36); if sac still present, counsel regarding D&C OR returning every 2 weeks for repeat ultrasound ←

INSTRUCTIONS FOR PATIENT
- Expect moderate (occasionally severe) cramping, bleeding and nausea
- Call or seek help if heavy bleeding (soaking 4 sanitary pads within 2 hours)
- Abstain from sexual intercourse, alcohol, and vitamins or folate supplements during treatment
- Either return for MIS or take it at home as directed
- Use acetaminophen or NSAIDs for analgesia; use codeine if inadequate relief
- Have a support person close by after MIS is given

PROBLEM MANAGEMENT
Pain
- Oral analgesics, including NSAIDs; 1/300 women needs parenteral analgesia *[Creinin, 1997]*

Bleeding
- D&C only for hemorrhage, or anemia requiring transfusion

Nausea/vomiting/diarrhea
- Rarely requires treatment; if needed, use antiemetics and Lomotil

FERTILITY AFTER USE
- Immediate return to baseline fertility. Contraceptive should be supplied immediately
- No evidence of harm in future pregnancies due to these medications

ELECTIVE MEDICAL ABORTION WITH MIFEPRISTONE (RU-486)(MIFEPREX) AND MISOPROSTOL (MIS)

FDA
APPROVAL
OCTOBER
2000

DESCRIPTION
- Mifepristone (200-600 mg) is administered first and acts as antiprogesterone to block ← continued support of pregnancy; 600 mg is approved dose
- Misoprostol is typically given 36-48 hours later to induce expulsion of the products of conception
- Used as abortifacient in France since 1989 and in other European countries and China. With some regimens, can be used up to 63 days gestation

EFFECTIVENESS
- Mifepristone alone 60-80% effective (200 mg is as effective as 600 mg) ←
- Mifepristone followed by MIS 92-98% effective

MECHANISMS

- Mifepristone blocks progesterone receptors and inhibits transcription, resulting in down-regulation of progesterone-dependent genes. This causes decidual necrosis and detachment of products of conception. Mifepristone also causes cervical softening
- Misoprostol induces uterine contractions and expulsion of pregnancy (may be taken either in the office or at home)

COST

- $100-300 for mifepristone plus additional costs

ADVANTAGES
Similar to methotrexate except:
- Can be more effective with certain regimens and generally is more rapid
- Can be used up to 63 days gestational age if misoprostol given vaginally

DISADVANTAGES
Similar to methotrexate except:
- Result not usually delayed
- May need to provide prolonged access to bathroom facilities if patients observed in office after misoprostol administration

COMPLICATIONS *[Silvestre, 1990]*
- Incomplete abortion (2%)
- Ongoing pregnancy (1%)
- Hemorrhage requiring emergency curettage (<1%)
- Blood transfusion (0.1%)
- Infection (0.1%)

CANDIDATES FOR USE
Similar to methotrexate candidates (p. 29) except:
- Gestational age up to 49 days if using oral misoprostol
- Gestational age up to 63 days if using vaginal misoprostol
- Not for use by chronic corticosteroid users

INITIATING METHOD
Similar to methotrexate (p. 29) except for protocol:
- *Day 1:* Mifepristone 600 mg orally (Mifeprex)
  Rh immunoglobulin if Rh negative
- *Day 3:* Give misoprostol (800 µg into posterior fornix of vagina or 400 µg orally)
  May observe patient 4 hrs; 44-70% of abortions occur in this time
- *Day 15:* Assess expulsion; pelvic exam, ultrasound (if needed)
  For an incomplete or failed abortion, perform D&C or offer observation and return appointment in 2-4 weeks

INSTRUCTIONS FOR PATIENT, PROBLEM MANAGEMENT, & FERTILITY AFTER USE
- Similar to methotrexate (p. 30)

EARLY MEDICAL ABORTION WITH MISOPROSTOL ALONE ◄——
Misoprostol is a prostaglandin analogue which causes very strong uterine contractions. More to follow in 2002-2003 book.

CHAPTER 12
Contraceptive Timing Issues - From the Old to the New
www.managingcontraception.com

Previous Timing Advice	Problems with Previous Advice	Better/New Advice
Start combined oral contraceptive pills (COCs) on Sunday of next menses (see case 1)	Pills less effective if started after first day of menses, backup needed	Start first day of menses or, if not pregnant, start today with backup
Case #1: 19 year-old is told to start COCs on Sunday of next cycle. However, her period starts on a Sunday. She is confused not knowing whether to start that day or in one week. If using the Sunday-start approach tell women that if next period begins on a Sunday, take first pill THAT DAY. If period begins any other day of the week take first pill the NEXT Sunday.		
Need periodic "rest" or "break" from COCs (see case 2)	Risk of pregnancy; Loss of noncontraceptive benefits Adds to myths about COC safety	No limit on duration of COC use Can use to menopause in healthy nonsmoking women
Case #2: To "take a break from pills," a 21 year-old student stops pills for the month her boyfriend will be away visiting the medical schools he is applying to. Plans change. He returns. They have intercourse and unintended pregnancy occurs. He is extremely supportive and is with her for abortion, but it is still extremely traumatic for her. Message: discourage brief "breaks" from taking pills.		
Must take 3 weeks of active pills and 1 week of (placebo pills) (see case 3)	Withdrawal bleeding not medically needed Menses cause some women medical problems and physical pain	Offer women with severe cyclic problems continuous COCs or make every cycle first day start to increase efficacy and avoid estrogen withdrawal symptoms
Case #3: 18 year-old has premenstrual irritability and depression each cycle. Switches from taking pills 21/7, 21/7, 21/7 to taking active pills for 84 days in a row followed by 7 days off. The number of episodes of PMS and depression may fall. (see page 104)		
Norplant/DMPA must be started during menses (see case 4)	Makes access much more difficult for some women	Insert/start anytime patient is not pregnant. If not near menses: DMPA – 7 days back up; Norplant – 3 days backup
Case #4: 20 year-old woman on COCs for 2 years. On day 10 of active pills. Told to return for Norplant insertion on next period. There is no reason to make her wait.		

Previous Timing Advice	Problems with Previous Advice	Better/New Advice
IUD must always be inserted during menses (see case 5)	Cramping worse; Expulsion rates higher Vaginal bleeding does NOT definitely exclude pregnancy Makes access much more difficult for some women	Insert any time in cycle when patient not pregnant. Midcycle best: lowest overall removal rate [White-1980]

Case #5: Condom breaks when couple has intercourse on day 13 of cycle, the day before her appointment to have IUD inserted. Told to return during next period. She does but she is pregnant. Could have received IUD at midcycle visit when it would have been an extremely effective postcoital contraceptive. (see pp 74-75, 77)

Previous Timing Advice	Problems with Previous Advice	Better/New Advice
Progestin methods (DMPA, Norplant) must wait until 6 weeks postpartum, especially breast-feeding women. Wait until 6 weeks postpartum before giving first Depo-Provera shot to breast-feeding women (see case 6)	Only women with anemia or strong history of postpartum depression may need delay. Breast feeding actually continues longer in DMPA users than non-users	Give first Depo-Provera injection to patient before she leaves the hospital (see p. 116)

Case #6: A 19 year-old woman who plans to breastfeed her baby is denied DMPA in the hospital after the delivery of her second child. She does not return for her 6-week PP exam after learning she will not see the same nurse midwife who delivered her baby. She was given an appointment several weeks later (now 8 or 9 weeks postpartum) so that she could see the same nurse midwife. By then, she was pregnant. Her postpartum visit turned out to be her first antepartum visit instead. After she delivered her third child (age 20), she again planned to nurse her baby. The policy was still not to give Depo-Provera to a lactating woman. The nurse midwife gave the woman her initial injection before she left the hospital.

Previous Timing Advice	Problems with Previous Advice	Better/New Advice
Place condom on erect penis (see case 7)	Early genital contact prior to condom placement allows STI transmission; Condom may never be placed	Apply condom before genital contact Partner's placement can cause erection

Case #7: 20 year-old man delays using condom until erection. Couple already have slippery fingers. They fumble around opening condom and trying to get it onto penis. Man's frustration is immense: he loses erection and has no orgasm! Frustration and loss of pleasure lead him to conclude that he will not consider using condoms in the future.

Previous Timing Advice	Problems with Previous Advice	Better/New Advice
Patients should seek EC after exposure (see case 8)	Early use of EC is more effective Pharmacies may not have EC on hand Access to clinics/centers on weekends/holidays limited	Advance prescription of EC should be offered to all at-risk women; Better yet, hand her the actual ECPs and instructions

Case #8: 20 year-old has prescription for either PLAN B (1+1) or Ovrette (20+20). Goes to 2 drugstores that have neither actually starting ECPs by 36 hours. If you are prescribing ECPs, you need to know which pharmacies in your vicinity actually carry the ECP you would like to prescribe

CHAPTER 13
Choosing Among Available Methods
www.managingcontraception.com/choices
www.plannedparenthood.org/library

THE BEST METHOD IS THE ONE USED EVERY TIME
THERE IS A METHOD FOR EVERY COUPLE
- Be aware of your own biases.
- Each contraceptive method has both advantages and disadvantages
- Effectiveness and safety are important (see Tables 13.2, p. 36 and 13.3, p. 37)
- Convenience and ability to use method may determine effectiveness
- Protection against STIs/HIV needs to be considered for women and men at risk
- Effects of method on menses may be very important to woman
- Ability to negotiate with partner may help determine method and selection
- Other influences (religion, privacy, past experience, friend's advice, frequency of intercourse) impact patient's preferences
- Discuss all methods with patient, even those you may not use in your own practice
- Consider discussing with couple, particularly if there appear to be issues ⬅

EFFECTIVENESS: measured by failure rates in 2 ways (see Table 13.2, p. 36)
Correct and consistent use first year failure rate: The percentage of women who become pregnant during their first year of use when they use the method correctly and consistently.
Typical use first year failure rates: The percentage of women who become pregnant during their first year of use. This number reflects the impact both of couples who use the method correctly and consistently and of those who do not. **This typical use failure rate is the relevant number to use when counseling new start users.**
- Failure rates may include previous users, restarters, or new starters

KEY QUESTIONS
- *Do you want to have any future pregnancies?*
  If she says no, be sure to offer sterilization in addition to the reversible methods
- *When (if ever) do you want to have your next child?*
  Helps teach need for preconceptional care and guides in selection of method.
- *What would you do if you had an accidental pregnancy?*
  Is abortion a viable backup for her?
- *What are you doing to protect yourself from STIs/AIDS?*
  Inclusion of counseling about safer sex practices and condoms may be critical considering:
- *What do you know about emergency contraception?*
  Would she like a package of ECPs or a prescription for ECPs?
- *Do you have any serious medical problems that could be adversely affected by a contraceptive?* ⬅
- *What contraceptive did you come to this office today wanting to use?* ⬅

TABLE 13.1 Comparative risk of unprotected intercourse on unintended pregnancies and STI infections*

Unintended pregnancy/coital act	PID per woman infected with cervical gonorrhea
17%-30% midcycle <1% during menses	40% if not treated 0% if promptly and adequately treated
Gonococcal transmission/coital act	**Tubal infertility per PID episode**
50% infected male, uninfected female 25% infected female, uninfected male	8% after first episode 20% after second episode 40% after three or more episodes

Cates W Jr. Reproductive tract infections. In: Hatcher RA, et al. Contraceptive Technology. 17th ed. New York: Ardent Media, 1998:181.

How is the contraceptive decision made? ◄

Most women who are currently using no method and come to a clinic or office to start contraception know exactly what method they want. Demographic and health surveys in 49 countries found in every country survey that 80 percent or more intending to use family planning came to a clinic knowing what method they wanted. In 26 of 49 surveys over 90% of women know what method they wanted to use. Only infrequently does a clinician need to deny a woman the contraceptive she wants. The World Health Organization's Medical Eligibility Criteria for Choosing a Contraceptive are summarized on pages A-1 to A-8 at the end of this book. These pages include an assessment of "the experts" on whether women with 90 to 100 conditions would be candidates of each contraceptive option. Study pages A-1 through A-8 well! While it is not always possible to give a woman the method she comes to you wanting, success tends to be greater if she is using the method she would like to use.

Table 13.2 Percentage of women experiencing an unintended pregnancy within the first year of typical use and the first year of perfect use and the percentage continuing use at the end of the first year: United States[*]

Method	% of Women Experiencing an Unintended Pregnancy within the First Year of Use		% of Women Continuing Use at One Year[1]
	Typical Use[2]	Perfect Use[3]	
Chance[4]	85	85	
Spermicides[5]	26	6	40
Periodic Abstinence			63
Calendar	25	9	
Ovulation Method	25	3	
Symptothermal[6]	25	2	
Post-ovulation	25	1	
Cervical Cap with spermicide			
Parous Women	40	26	42
Nulliparous Women	20	9	56
Sponge			
Parous Women	40	20	42
Nulliparous Women	20	9	56
Diaphragm with spermicide[7]	20	6	56
Withdrawal	19	4	
Condom without spermicide[8]			
Reality Female Polyurethane condom	21	5	56
Male (Latex or polyurethane)	14	3	61
Pill			
Progestin only	5	0.5	
Combined	5	0.1	
IUD			
Progesterone-releasing	2.0	1.5	81
Copper	0.8	0.6	78
Levonorgestrel-releasing	0.1	0.1	81
Progestin injections	0.3	0.3	42[11]
Combined hormone injections	0.2	0.1	
Levonorgestrel-releasing implants	0.05	0.05	88
Female Sterilization	0.5	0.5	100
Male Sterilization	0.15	0.10	100

Emergency Contraceptive Pills: Treatment with COCs initiated within 72 hours after unprotected intercourse reduces the risk of pregnancy by at least 60-75%. Pregnancy rates lower if initiated in first 12 hours. [10] Progestin-only EC reduces pregnancy risk by 85%.

Lactational Amenorrhea Method: LAM is a highly effective, temporary method of contraception.[11]

[1] Among couples attempting to avoid pregnancy, the percentage who continue to use a method for 1 year

[2] Among typical couples who initiate use of a method (not necessarily for the first time), the percentage who experience an accidental pregnancy during the first year if they do not stop use for any other reason

[3] Among couples who initiate use of a method (not necessarily for the first time) and who use it perfectly (both consistently and correctly), the percentage who experience an accidental pregnancy during the first year if they do not stop use for any other reason

[4] The percentages becoming pregnant in columns 2 and 3 are based on data from populations where contraception is not used and from women who cease using contraception in order to become pregnant. Among such populations, about 89% become pregnant within 1 year. This estimate was lowered slightly (to 85) to represent the percentages who would become pregnant within 1 year among women now relying on reversible methods of contraception if they abandoned contraception altogether

[5] Foams, creams, gels, vaginal suppositories, and vaginal film

[6] Cervical mucus (ovulation) method supplemented by calendar in the pre-ovulatory and basal body temperature in the post-ovulatory phases

[7] With spermicidal cream or jelly

[8] Without spermicides

[9] The median one-year continuation rate for 10 studies in the 1990s was 42%

[10] The treatment schedule is one dose within 72 hours after unprotected intercourse, and a second dose 12 hours after the first dose. See page 70 for pills that may be used

[11] However, to maintain effective protection against pregnancy, another method of contraception must be used as soon as menstruation resumes, the frequency or duration of breast-feedings is reduced, bottle feeds are introduced, or the baby reaches 6 months of age

[*] Trussell J, Kowal D. The essentials of contraception. In: Hatcher RA, et al. *Contraceptive Technology*, 17th ed. New York: Ardent Media, 1998:216-7. Slight adaptations from CT table.

Table 13.3 Major methods of contraception and some related safety concerns, side effects, and noncontraceptive benefits
*Trussell J, Kowal D. The essentials of contraception. In Hatcher RA, et al. *Contraceptive Technology*. 17th ed. New York: Ardent Media, 1998:235. Slight adaptations from CT table.

METHOD	DANGERS	SIDE EFFECTS	NONCONTRACEPTIVE BENEFITS*
COC pill and combined injection	Cardiovascular complications, (DVT, PE, MI, hypertension), depression, hepatic adenoma, slight increase in adenocarcinoma of cervix and breast cancer risk	Nausea, vomiting, headaches, dizziness, mastalgia, chloasma, spotting and bleeding, mood changes including, rarely, severe depression	Decreases menstrual pain, PMS, and blood loss; protects against symptomatic PID requiring hospitalization, ovarian and endometrial carcinomas, some benign tumors (leiomyomata, benign breast masses), ectopic pregnancies and ovarian cysts; reduces acne; Injection has demonstrated cycle control only
Progestin-only pills	None	Spotting, breakthrough bleeding, amenorrhea, mood changes, headaches, hot flashes	Lactation not disturbed. Decreased menstrual pain & blood loss
Progestin-only implants	Infection at implant site, reaction to anesthesia, complicated removal, depression	Menstrual changes, mood changes, weight gain or loss, headaches, hair loss	Lactation not disturbed. Less blood loss per cycle. Reduced risk of ectopic pregnancy
Progestin-only injections	Allergic reaction, possible weight gain, glucose intolerance, depression	Menstrual changes, weight gain, headaches, hair loss, adverse impact on lipids, mood changes including, rarely, severe depression	Lactation not disturbed. Reduces risk of sickle cell crises, reduces risk of endometrial cancer, ovarian cysts, mittelschmerz. May reduce risk of PID, ovarian cancer
IUD	PID following insertion, uterine perforation, hemorrhage with expulsion	Copper-IUD increases menstrual flow, blood loss and cramping; LNg IUD may cause irregular bleeding/amenorrhea	Copper T and Levonorgestrel IUDs reduce risk for ectopic pregnancies. Levonorgestrel IUD dramatically reduces menstrual bleeding, cramping and pain
Sterilization	Surgical complications, hemorrhage, infection, organ damage, anesthetic complications, ectopic pregnancy	Pain at surgical site, adhesion formation, subsequent regret	Women: reduced risk of ovarian cancer, endometrial cancer, ectopic pregnancy, PID Men: none known
Abstinence	None known	None except possible peer pressure; Partner may become sexually active	Prevents STIs, cervical dysplasia; enhanced self-image possible
Male latex condom	Anaphylactic reaction to latex (use polyurethane)	Decrease spontaneity or sensation; allergic reaction to latex	Reduces risk of STIs, and cervical dysplasia
Female condom	TSS (no cases)	Difficult to use, vaginal and bladder infection, allergy to spermicide	May reduce STI and cervical dysplasia risk
Diaphragm Cervical cap	TSS, anaphylactic reaction to latex	Vaginal and bladder infection, vaginal erosions from poorly fit device, allergy to spermicide/latex	Reduces risk of cervical STIs, PID and possibly cervical dysplasia

CHAPTER 14
Abstinence

DESCRIPTION
Surveys have revealed a wide variety of opinions about what constitutes sexual activity. However, from a family planning perspective, the definition of abstinence is clear, it is the absence of genital contact that could permit a pregnancy i.e. penile penetration into the vagina. Some authors argue that abstinence is not a form of contraception, but is a lifestyle choice because an abstinent person is not having sex and, therefore, needs no contraception. Regardless, abstinence is promoted as a means of reducing unintended pregnancies.

EFFECTIVENESS
Perfect use failure rate in first year: 0%
Typical use failure rates in first year: Higher due to changes in priorities and practices.

MECHANISM
Sperm excluded from female reproductive tract, which prevents fertilization

COST: None

ADVANTAGES
Menstrual: none
Sexual/psychological:
• Can increase self esteem and positive self image if woman and man morally values it
Cancers, tumors, and masses:
• Risk of cervical dysplasia far less if no vaginal intercourse has occurred
Other:
• Reduces risk of STIs (varies by what other sexual practices involved)
• Can be started at any time
• Many religions and cultures endorse (at least at some time in the woman's life)

DISADVANTAGES
Menstrual: None
Sexual/psychological:
• Frustration or sense of rejection if abstinence not self-selected
Cancers, tumors, and masses: None except indirectly. Virgins who remain nulliparous have an increased risk for breast and ovarian cancer (but decreased risk for cervical cancer)
Other:
• Requires commitment and self control; partner may seek other partner(s)
• Patient and her partner may not be prepared to contracept if they stop abstaining

COMPLICATIONS
• No medical complications
• Patient may be in situations where she/he would like to abstain, but her/his partner does not agree. Women have been raped and beaten for refusing to have intercourse. Clearly this is wrong. However, occasionally there can be dire consequences of the decision not to have intercourse

CANDIDATES FOR USE

- Individuals or couples who feel they have ability to refrain from sexual intercourse

Adolescents:
- Very appropriate method but need to learn negotiating skills to effectively use abstinence and information about contraceptive methods for future
- Counseling may also include discussions on masturbation and "outercourse" (alternative ways of expressing affection/attraction/sexuality with partner)

INITIATING METHOD

- Provide negotiating skills, how to say no, and how to resist peer (societal) pressures
- Recommend that patient ensure that partner explicitly agrees to abstain
- Can return to abstinence at any time in life

INSTRUCTIONS FOR PATIENT

- Establish ground rules for herself and partner
- Prepare for time when (or if) decision to stop abstaining arises, provide contraceptive counseling now
- Have condoms and emergency contraception on hand in case of need

PROBLEM MANAGEMENT

Partner does not want to abstain:
- Provide counseling in negotiating skills; consider couple counseling
- Provide counseling in other forms of sexual pleasuring if patient interested (masturbation or outercourse)
- Seriously consider another birth control method

FERTILITY AFTER USE

- Protects against upper reproductive tract infection preserving woman's fertility
- Patient's baseline fertility (ability to cause pregnancy or become pregnant) is not altered if patient decides to have intercourse

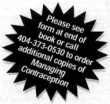

Please see form at end of book or call 404-373-0530 to order additional copies of Managing Contraception

Now available in Spanish as well as English

DESCRIPTION

In general, breast-feeding delays the return of fertility postpartum. However, LAM is an effective method only under specific conditions:

- Woman breast-feeding exclusively; both day and night feedings (at least 90% of baby's nutrition derived from breast-feeding)
- The woman is amenorrheic (spotting which occurs in the first 56 days postpartum is not regarded as menses)
- The infant is less than 6 months old

In the U.S., the median duration of breast-feeding is approximately 3 months. It is wise to provide a woman with another method to use when she no longer fulfills all the conditions

EFFECTIVENESS *(Kennedy, 1998)*

Perfect use failure rate in first 6 months: 0.5%
Typical use failure rate in first 6 months: 2%

At any time a woman is concerned, emergency contraception may be used by a nursing mother (preferably with Levonorgestrel-only pills)

MECHANISM

Baby suckling on the mother's nipples causes a surge in maternal prolactin, which inhibits estrogen production and ovulation

COST: None

ADVANTAGES

NOTE: Most advantages and disadvantages are attributable to breast-feeding itself. The additional benefits accruing to LAM as a contraceptive method are minimal

Menstrual: Involution of the uterus occurs more rapidly; suppresses menses

Sexual/psychological: Breast-feeding pleasurable to some women
- Facilitates bonding between mother and child (if not stressful)

Cancers, tumors, and masses: Reduces risk of ovarian cancer; possible slight protective effect against breast cancer

Other:
- Can be used immediately after childbirth
- Provides the healthiest food for baby
- Protects baby against asthma, allergies, URIs and diarrhea by passage of mother's antibodies into breastmilk
- Facilitates postpartum weight loss
- Less expensive and less time preparing bottles and feedings

DISADVANTAGES

Menstrual: Return to menses unpredictable

Sexual/psychological:
- Breast-feeding may be embarrassing to mother
- Hypoestrogenism of breast-feeding may cause dyspareunia due to lack of lubrication
- Woman may be self conscious about breasts leaking during lovemaking
- Tender breasts may decrease sexual pleasure

Cancers, tumors, and masses: None

Other:
- Effectiveness after 6 months is markedly reduced; return to fertility can precede menses
- Frequent breast-feeding may be inconvenient or perceived as inconvenient

- No protection against STIs, HIV, AIDS
- If the mother is HIV+, there is a 14%-29% chance that HIV will be passed to infant via breast milk. Antiretroviral therapy decreases risk of transmission
- Sore nipples and breasts; risk of mastitis associated with breast-feeding

COMPLICATIONS: Mastitis risk increases

CANDIDATES FOR USE
- Amenorrheic women less then 6 months postpartum who breast-feed their babies exclusively
- Women free of a blood born infection which could be passed to the newborn
- Women not on drugs which can adversely affect their babies
- Adolescents may find this method difficult

MEDICAL ELIGIBILITY CHECKLIST
Ask the patient the questions below. If she answers "NO" to ALL questions, she can use LAM. If she answers Yes to any questions, follow the instructions. Sometimes there is a way to incorporate LAM into her contraceptive plans; in other situations, LAM is contraindicated.

1. Is your baby 6 months old or older?

☐ No ☐ Yes   Help her choose another method to bolster the contraceptive effect of LAM.

2. Has your menstrual period returned? (Bleeding in the first 8 weeks after childbirth does not count)

☐ No ☐ Yes   After 8 weeks postpartum, if a woman has 2 straight days of menstrual bleeding, or her menstrual period has returned, she can no longer count on LAM as her contraceptive. Help her choose another method.

3. Have you begun to breast-feed less often? Do you regularly give the baby other food or liquid (other than water)?

☐ No ☐ Yes   If the baby's feeding pattern has just changed, explain that patient must fully or nearly fully breast-feed around the clock to protect against pregnancy. If she is not fully or nearly fully breast-feeding, she cannot use LAM effectively. Help her choose another method.

4. Has a health-care provider told you not to breast-feed your baby?

☐ No ☐ Yes   If a patient is not breast-feeding, she cannot use LAM. Help her choose another method. A woman should not breast-feed if she is taking mood altering recreational drugs, reserpine, ergotamine, antimetabolites, cyclosporine, bromocriptine, tetracycline, radioactive drugs, lithium, or certain anticoagulants (heparin and coumadin are safe); if her baby has a specific infant metabolic disorder; or possibly if she carries viral hepatitis or is HIV positive. All others can and should consider breast-feeding for the health benefits to the infant. In 1997, the FDA advised the manufacturer of Prozac (fluoxetine) to revise its labeling; it now states that "nursing while on Prozac is not recommended." On the other hand, Briggs notes that "the authors of a 1996 review stated that they encouraged women to continue breast-feeding while taking the drug [Nulman Tetralogy - 1996][Briggs - 1998]

5. Are you infected with HIV, the virus that causes AIDS?

☐ No ☐ Yes   Where other infectious diseases kill many babies, mothers should be encouraged to breast-feed. HIV, however, may be passed to the baby in breast milk. When infectious diseases are a low risk and there is safe, affordable food for the baby, advise her to feed her baby that other food. Help her choose a birth control method other than LAM. A meta-analysis of published prospective trials estimated the risk of transmission of HIV with breast-feeding is 14% if the mother was infected prenatally but is 29% if woman has her primary infection in the post partum period.

41

***6. Do you know how long you plan to breast-feed your baby before you start
supplementing his/her diet?***

   ☐ No   ☐ Yes   In the U.S. the median duration of breast-feeding is approximately
3 months. Often breast-feeding women do not know when their menses will return, when
they will start supplementing breast-feeding with other foods or exactly when they will stop
breast-feeding their infant. It is wise to provide a woman with the contraceptive she will
use when the answer to one of the above questions becomes positive and with a backup
contraceptive and ECPs even during the period when breast-feeding is effective.

INITIATING METHOD
- Patient should start exclusively breast-feeding immediately after delivery
- Ensure that woman is breast-feeding fully or almost fully (>90% of baby's feedings);
  feedings around the clock
- Encourage use of second method of contraception if any questions about LAM effectiveness

INSTRUCTIONS FOR PATIENT
- Breast-feed consistently and correctly for maximum effectiveness
- Breast milk should constitute at least 90% of baby's feedings

PROBLEM MANAGEMENT
Deficient milk supply:
- Commonly caused by insufficient nursing, use of artificial nipple, fatigue or maternal stress
- Encourage woman to breast-feed often (8-10 times daily), eat well, get additional rest,
  drink lots of fluids and take prenatal vitamins and iron supplements
- Immediately postpartum women should breast-feed every 2-3 hours
- Estrogen-containing contraceptives

Sore nipples:
- Provide good support
- Commonly caused by incorrect positioning of the baby to the breast or infection
- Check for correct ways of latching and suckling; be sure to break the suction before
  removing the baby from the breast
- Improve with practice; changing the baby's position for feeding, which will change the
  pressure points on the nipple may help
- Allow nipples to air dry with breast milk on the areola to reduce infection and nipple ◄
  soreness
- Do not cleanse breasts other than water in shower
- Applying lanolin to nipples after each feeding may decrease soreness ◄

Sore breasts:
- Apply heat on sore areas; some women apply teabag as compress on sore nipples
- Nurse frequently or use pump to get excess milk out of affected breast
- Encourage additional rest
- Seek medical evaluation if any erythema, fever or other signs or symptoms of infection
  develop

Other:
- Stress, fear, lack of confidence, lack of strong desire to succeed at breast feeding, lack of
  partner and/or societal support, and/or poor nutrition can cause problems

FERTILITY AFTER USE
Patient's baseline fertility (ability to become pregnant) is not altered once patient
discontinues breast-feeding.

TEN STEPS TO SUCCESSFUL BREAST-FEEDING ◀

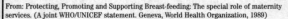

From: Protecting, Promoting and Supporting Breast-feeding: The special role of maternity services. (A joint WHO/UNICEF statement. Geneva, World Health Organization, 1989)

All healthcare facilities where childbirth is undertaken should:

1. Have a written breast-feeding policy that is routinely communicated to all health care staff.
2. Train all health care staff in skills necessary to implement this policy.
3. Inform all pregnant women about the benefits and management of breast-feeding.
4. Help mothers initiate breast-feeding within the first 30 minutes after birth.
5. Show mothers how to breast-feed and how to maintain lactation even if they should be separated from their infants because of a medical reason.
6. Give newborn infants no milk feeds or water other than breast milk unless indicated for a medical reason.
7. Allow mothers and infants to remain together 24 hours a day from birth.
8. Encourage natural breast-feeding on demand.
9. Do not give, or encourage the use of artificial teats or dummies to breast-fed infants.
10. Promote the establishment of breast-feeding support groups and refer mothers to these on discharge from the hospital or clinic.

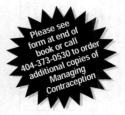

Please see form at end of book or call 404-373-0530 to order additional copies of Managing Contraception

All breast-feeding women should be provided contraception because:
- Duration of breast-feeding in the U.S. is typically brief
- Most couples resume intercourse a few weeks after delivery
- Spacing of pregnancies is important to maternal and child health
- Ovulation may precede first menses

Table 16.1 *When to initiate contraception in breast-feeding women:*

METHOD	WHEN TO START IN LACTATING WOMEN	EFFECT ON BREAST MILK
Condoms (Male & Female), Sponge	• Immediately after lochia stops (intercourse prior to that time carries risk of infection)	No effect
Cervical Cap, Diaphragm	• 4-6 weeks postpartum, after cervix and vagina normalized	No effect
Progestin-Only Methods • Depo-Provera • Progestin - Only Pills • Norplant	• Most authorities, including National Medical Committee of the Planned Parenthood Federation of America, consider it appropriate to initiate any progestin-only method immediately postpartum • WHO and International Planned Parenthood Federation recommend waiting 6 weeks postpartum. Concern about adequate maternal nutrition may be important consideration in developing countries	• No significant impact on milk quality or production • Breast-feeding prolonged • Breast fed children of DMPA users grow at normal rate
Combined Pills or Combined Injections	• American Academy of Pediatrics recommends use when infant's diet supplemented but no sooner than 3-6 weeks postpartum • Most conservative position: await weaning	Quality and quantity of breast milk may be diminished if used prior to establishment of lactation. After establishment, COCs have no significant impact on lactation
IUD: • Copper, • Progesterone • Levonorgestrel	• May insert within first 20 minutes after delivery of placenta with special equipment • Perforation rates at insertion may be higher in breast-feeding women	No effect
Tubal Sterilization	Usually done in first 24-48 hours postpartum, or await complete uterine involution for interval tubal sterilization (> 6 weeks postpartum)	No effect

CHAPTER 17

Natural Family Planning (NFP) & Fertility Awareness Methods (FAM)

www.dml.georgetown.edu/depts/irh OR www.usc.edu/hsc/info/newman/resource/nfp.html

DESCRIPTION

Uses physical signs, symptoms, and cycle data to determine when ovulation occurs. Same techniques may be used to help couples become pregnant by detecting ovulation. When couples use NFP, they abstain from intercourse during the at-risk fertile days. With FAM, couples use another method such as barriers or withdrawal during those days. Perhaps we should ← be more proactive in urging fertility awareness as complementary to all contraceptive methods Techniques used to determine high-risk fertile days include:

1. Calendar Method

- Record days of menses prospectively for 6 cycles
- Most estimates assume that sperm can survive 2-3 days and ovulation occurs 14 days before menses (motile sperm have been found as long as 7 days after intercourse and the extreme ← interval following a single act of coitus leading to an achieved pregnancy is 6 days *[Speroff 1999]*)
- Earliest day of fertile period = day # in a cycle corresponding to **shortest cycle length minus 18**
- Latest day of fertile period = day # in a cycle corresponding to **longest cycle length minus 11**

2. Cervical Mucus Ovulation Detection Method

- Women check quantity and character of mucus on the vulva or introitus with fingers or tissue paper each day for several months to learn cycle:
  - Post-menstrual mucus: scant or undetectable
  - Pre-ovulation mucus: cloudy, yellow or white, sticky
  - Ovulation mucus: clear, wet, sticky (but slippery)
  - Post-ovulation fertile mucus: thick, cloudy, sticky
  - Post-ovulation post-fertile mucus: scant or undetectable
- When using method during preovulatory period, must abstain 24 hours after intercourse to make test interpretable
- Abstinence or barrier method through fertile period
- Intercourse without restriction beginning on the 4th day after the last day of wet, clear, slippery mucus

3. Basal Body Temperature Method (BBT)

- Assumes that early morning temperature measured before arising will increase noticeably (0.4-0.8° F) with ovulation; fertile period is defined as the day of the first temperature drop or first elevation through 3 consecutive days of elevated temperature

4. Post-ovulation Method

- Permits unprotected intercourse only after signs of ovulation have subsided

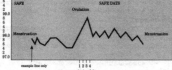

Figure 17.1 Basal body temperature variations during a menstrual cycle

5. Symptothermal Method

- Combines at least two methods — usually cervical mucus changes with BBT
- May also include Mittelschmerz, change in libido, and changes in cervical texture, position and dilation to detect ovulation
  - During preovulatory and ovulatory periods, cervix softens, opens and is moister
  - During postovulatory period, cervix drops, becomes firm and closes

45

In my view, with any combination of present technologies, only the second infertile phase should be relied on by a woman who feels that she must avoid pregnancy. The first phase is only suitable for those who are delaying a wanted prenancy ('spacing'). The one exception to this recommendation might be a woman with very regular longish menstrual cycles (never less than 28 days) who is good at detecting mucus and cervical changes. She should abstain in each cycle from the first day of detection of mucus or from 20 days before her shortest cycle would end, whichever comes earlier, to identify the first potentially fertile day. *[Guillebaud - 1999]* ◄━━━

EFFECTIVENESS (see Table 13.2, page 36)

NFP/FAM First-year failure rate (100 women-years of use)

Method	Typical use*	Perfect use
Calendar	25	9
Ovulation Method	25	3
Symptothermal	25	2
Post-ovulation	25	1

*FAM usually more effective than NFP   *[Trussell in Contraceptive Technology, 1998]*

MECHANISM: Abstinence or barriers during fertile period

COST: Training, supplies (special digital basal body thermometer or another thermometer), and barriers

ADVANTAGES
Menstrual:
- No change
- Helps woman learn more about her menstrual physiology

Sexual/psychological: Men and women can work together in using this method
Cancers, tumors, and masses: None
Other:
- May be only method acceptable to couples for cultural or religious reasons
- Helps couples achieve pregnancy when practiced in reverse

DISADVANTAGES
Menstrual:
- Difficult to use in early adolescence when approaching menopause and in postpartum women when cycles are irregular (or absent) or with vaginal infections

Sexual/psychological:
- Requires abstinence, barrier method, or another contraceptive that does not change pattern of ovulation during 6-12 month learning/data-gathering period
- Complete abstinence in anovulatory cycle, if using post-ovulation techniques
- Requires discipline, good communication and full commitment of both partners
- Requires abstinence at time of ovulation, which is the time of peak libido

Cancers, tumors, and masses: None
Other:
- May not be helpful during time of stress
- Method very unforgiving of improper use
- Does not protect against STIs
- Relatively high failure rate

COMPLICATIONS

None; no increased risk of birth defects, spontaneous abortion or chromosomal abnormalities seen in women who conceive from "aged gametes" using NFP correctly

CANDIDATES FOR USE

• Women with regular, predictable menstrual cycles
• Those with religious/cultural proscriptions against using other methods
• Those meeting medical eligibility criteria
• Highly motivated couples willing to commit to extensive abstinence or to use barriers during vulnerable periods

Adolescents: Not appropriate until regular menstrual cycles established

MEDICAL ELIGIBILITY CHECKLIST

Ask the woman the questions below. If she answers NO to ALL questions, she CAN use any fertility awareness-based method if she wants. If she answers YES to any question, follow the instructions. No conditions restrict use of these methods, but some conditions can make them harder to use effectively.

1. Do you have a medical condition that would make pregnancy especially dangerous?

☐ No ☐ Yes She may want to choose a more effective method. If not, stress careful use of fertility awareness-based methods to avoid pregnancy and availability of EC

2. Do you have irregular or prolonged menstrual cycles? Vaginal bleeding between periods?
For younger women: Are your periods just starting?
For older women: Have your periods become irregular, or have they stopped?

☐ No ☐ Yes Predicting her fertile time with only the calendar method may be hard or impossible. She can use basal body temperature (BBT) and/or cervical mucus, or she may prefer another method

3. Did you recently give birth or have an abortion? Are you breast-feeding?
Do you have any other condition that affects menstrual bleeding, such as stroke, serious liver disease, hypothyroidism or hyperthyroidism, or cervical cancer?

☐ No ☐ Yes These conditions may affect fertility signs, making fertility awareness-based methods hard to use. For this reason, a woman or couple may prefer a different method. If not, they may need more counseling and follow-up to use the method effectively

4. Do you have any infections or diseases that may change cervical mucus, basal body temperatures, or menstrual bleeding—such as sexually transmitted disease (STD) or pelvic inflammatory disease (PID) in the last 3 months, or vaginal infection?

☐ No ☐ Yes These conditions may affect fertility signs, making fertility awareness-based methods hard to use. Once an infection is treated and reinfection is avoided, however, a woman can use fertility awareness-based methods more easily

5. If you recently stopped using Depo-Provera or OCs, are your periods still irregular?

☐ No ☐ Yes If her cycles have not been re-established, she may prefer to use another method until cycles are regular

INITIATING METHOD

- Requires several months of data collection and analysis
- Description of methods
- Formal training necessary. Couples may be trained together
- Resources are available from:
  1. Calgary Billings Centre of Natural Family Planning, Room 1, 1247 Bel-Aire Dr SW, Calgary, AB T2V 2C1, (403) 252-3929, www.billings-centre.ab.ca
  2. California Association of Natural Family Planning, 1010 - 11th St, Suite 200, Sacramento, CA 95814, (877) 332-2637, www.canfp.org
  3. The Couple to Couple League International, PO Box 111184, Cincinnati, OH 45211-1184, (513) 471-2000, www.ccli.org
  4. Institute for Reproductive Health, Georgetown University Medical Center, 3 PHC, Room 300r, 3800 Reservoir Rd, NW, Washington, DC 20007, (202) 687-1392, www.dml.georgetown.edu/depts/irh
  5. National Center for Women's Health, Pope Paul VI Institute, 6901 Mercy Road, Omaha, NE 68106-2604, (402) 390-6600, www.popepaulvi.com
  6. Family of the Americas Foundation, Inc., PO Box 1170, Dunkirk, MD 20754-1170, (800) 443-3395, www.familyplanning.net
  7. Northwest Family Services, 4805 NE Glisan St, Portland, OR 97213, (503) 230-6377, www.nwfs.org
  8. Twin Cities NFP Center, HealthEast, St. Joseph's Hospital, 69 W Exchange St, St. Paul, MN 55102, (651) 232-3088, www.tcnfp.org

INSTRUCTIONS FOR PATIENT

- Requires discipline, communication, listening skills, full commitment of both partners
- If using FAM, use contraception during fertile days
- If using NFP, abstain from sexual intercourse during fertile days

FOLLOW-UP

- Have you had sexual intercourse during "unsafe" times during your cycle?
- Discuss use of emergency contraception if having sex during "unsafe" times during cycle

PROBLEM MANAGEMENT

Inconsistent use and risk taking: Educate about emergency contraception when women start using method

FERTILITY AFTER USING

- Return to baseline fertility

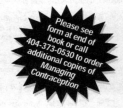

Please see form at end of book or call 404-373-0530 to order additional copies of Managing Contraception

DESCRIPTION

Condoms for men are sheaths made of latex, polyurethane or natural membranes (usually lamb cecum), which are placed over the penis prior to genital contact and worn until after ejaculation. Latex condoms are available in at least 2 sizes, in a wide variety of textures and thicknesses (0.03-0.09 mm), and come with or without spermicidal coating. Two brands of polyurethane condoms are currently available in the US. Both latex and polyurethane are impermeable to bacteria and viruses and offer a significant reduction in the spread of STIs with consistent and correct use. Natural membrane condoms may not provide that additional STI protection. Condoms may be used as a primary contraceptive method, as a back-up method, or with another method to provide STI prevention. **When used as a primary method, it is recommended that condoms be coupled with advance provision/prescription of emergency contraceptive pills (ECPs)**

EFFECTIVENESS [Trussell J in Contraceptive Technology, 1998]

Perfect use failure rate in the first year of use: 3% (See Table 13.2, page 36)
Typical use failure rate in the first year of use: 14%
- Comparative testing has shown that latex and polyurethane condoms provide the same pregnancy protection. However, there was a significant difference between the materials in slippage and breakage rates:

Condom Breakage and Slippage	Polyurethane	Latex
Trial 1	10.5%	1.7%
Trial 2	8.5%	1.6%

MECHANISM

- Condoms act as a mechanical barrier; they prevent pregnancy by preventing the passage of sperm into the female reproductive tract.
- Sheathing the shaft of the penis and trapping the ejaculate also reduces transmission and acquisition of bacterial and viral STIs, including HIV.
- It has not been determined whether a spermicidal condom increases either the contraceptive efficacy or the STI protection compared to a nonspermicidal condom (see statement from CDC STI Treatment Guidelines on page 145 of this book)

COST

- Average retail cost for latex condoms is $0.50, but some designer condoms cost several dollars. Polyurethane condoms cost $.80-$2.00 each
- Public entities often offer free condoms. Purchasers of large numbers of condoms may buy condoms for as low as 4 to 6 cents per condom
- The spermicide-coated latex condoms are not necessarily more expensive, but their average shelf life is reduced to 2 years (depending on the manufacturer) compared to the 5-year shelf life for unmedicated latex condoms.

ADVANTAGES

Menstrual: No impact on menses per se, but couple may feel more comfortable having intercourse during menses if a condom is used

Sexual/psychological:
- Intercourse may be more pleasurable because fear of pregnancy and STIs is decreased
- Some men may maintain erection longer with condoms, making sex more enjoyable
- If the woman puts the condom on, it may add to sexual pleasure
- Male involvement is encouraged as it is essential!
- Availability of wide selection of condom types and designs can add variety
- Makes sex less messy for women by catching the ejaculate

Cancers/tumors and masses:

- Decrease in HPV transmission may decrease risk of cervical dysplasia/cancer and external genital warts
- Decrease in HIV transmission reduces risks of AIDS-related malignancies

Other:

- Readily available over the counter; no medical visit required
- Usually inexpensive for single use
- Easily transportable (eg, between 2 photos in wallet; but don't leave in wallet too long; probably ok for 2 months) ←
- Opportunity for couples to improve communication and negotiating skills
- Immediately active after placement
- Significantly reduces risk of HIV transmission (Figure 18.2, p. 54) and some other STIs
- May reduce risk of PID and subsequent infertility, ectopic pregnancy and chronic pelvic pain by reducing risk of cervicitis

DISADVANTAGES

Menstrual: None

Sexual/psychological:

- Use may interrupt or be perceived as interrupting lovemaking. Requires discipline to resist impulse to progress to intercourse after erection
- May cause man to lose erection
- Blunting of sensation or "unnatural" feeling with intercourse
- Plain condoms may decrease lubrication and provide less stimulation for woman (use water-based lubricant if this is a problem)
- Requires prompt withdrawal after ejaculation, which may decrease pleasure for woman
- Makes sex messier for the man

Cancers/tumors and masses: None

Other:

- Requires education/experience for successful use
- Either member of couple may have latex allergy or reaction to spermicide (polyurethane condom is appropriate alternative)
- Users must avoid petroleum-based vaginal products when using latex condoms (Figure 18.1, p. 53) (polyurethane condoms appropriate alternative)
- Couples may be embarrassed to purchase or to apply condoms due to taboos about touching genitalia

COMPLICATIONS

- Allergic reactions to latex may be life threatening; 2-3% of Americans (men and women) have a latex allergy; up to 14% of latex workers are latex sensitive
- Condom retained in vagina (uncommon) exposes woman to risk of infection as well as pregnancy. If this occurs: 1. try to remove by pinching with second and third fingers or 2. enlist partner's help or 3. go to clinician ASAP and 4. consider EC.

PRESCRIBING PRECAUTIONS

- Men who are unable to maintain erection when they wear condoms
- Men with abnormal ejaculatory pathways not sheathed by condom
- Woman whose partners will not use condoms
- Women who require high contraceptive efficacy should, at a minimum, add another method in addition to the condom
- Couples in which either partner has latex allergy should avoid latex condoms (can use Durex, Avanti, Trojan-Supra, or Reality female condom)
- Couples in which either partner has spermicide allergy should avoid spermicide-coated condoms

CANDIDATES FOR USE

- Most couples can use condoms except, sometimes, those listed in PRESCRIBING PRECAUTIONS
- May be used alone or coupled with a second contraceptive method for enhanced pregnancy protection or disease prevention

Special applications for infection control:
- Non-monogamous couples, during pregnancy as well as at all other times ◄——
- New partners
- After delivery or loss to reduce risk of endometritis
- Couples with known viral infections (HIV, HPV, HSV) in areas sheathed by device

Adolescents: Excellent option, especially when combined with another method and/or routinely using ECPs as backup

INITIATING METHOD

Couples desiring to use condoms often benefit from concrete instructions. Use a model and actual condom. Counsel new users about:
- Options among condom types
- Storage for safety and ready access
- How to negotiate condom use with partner
- When to place condom
- How to open package and place correct side of condom over penis
- How to unroll and allow space for ejaculate (depending on condom design)
- How to handle mishaps

Provide ECPs to couples relying on the condom for birth control to insure immediate use after condom failure. This will minimize risk of unintended pregnancy risk.

INSTRUCTIONS FOR PATIENTS (See Figure 18.1, pg. 53)

- Learn how to use a condom long before you need it. Both women and men need to know how. Practice with models (bananas) or man's penis
- Buy condoms in advance and carry with you to prevent detection and puncture
- Keep extra condoms out of sunlight and heat which might weaken latex condoms
- Try new condoms to find favorite size and texture and to add variety
- Check date on condom carefully. It may be an expiration date OR a date of production. ◄——
  If it is an expiration date, do not use beyond expiration date. If it is a date of production, condom may be used for several years from the date of production (3 years for spermicidal condoms, 5 years for nonspermicidal latex condoms)
- Open package carefully and squeeze condom out. Avoid tearing condom with fingernails, foil wrapping, teeth, rings, etc.
- Use appropriate water-based lubricant (see page 53) Never put lubricant inside the condom
- Place condom over penis before any genital contact. Either partner can put it on!
- Consider placing a second condom (larger size) over lubricated condom if history of previous breakage or if man has any evidence of STI or desires enhanced sensation
- If condom used for oral or rectal intercourse (which is not recommended by manufacturers), replace condom prior to vaginal entry
- Vigorous sex can be fun but can break the condom. Consider using 2 condoms ◄——
- Immediately after ejaculation (before loss of erection) hold rim of condom against shaft of penis and remove condom-covered penis from vagina
- Remove condom from the penis and check for any breaks
- Dispose of condom. Do not reuse
- If a condom falls off, slips, tears or breaks, apply vaginal spermicidal foam immediately and start using ECPs as soon as possible. If you do not have ECPs, call 1-888-NOT-2-LATE or check www.not-2-late.com to find out how to get them. If any risk for STIs, seek medical care

FOLLOW-UP

- Are you and your partner comfortable using condoms?
- Have you had any problems with using the condom? Breaking? Slipping off? Decreased sensation? Vaginal soreness with use? Skin irritation or redness during the day after using it?
- Have you had any post-coital "yeast infection" symptoms? (A woman may confuse an allergic reaction to the condom and/or spermicide with a candidal infection)
- Have you had intercourse—even once—without a condom?
- Did you have any problems with ECPs?
- Do you need more ECPs?
- When do you plan to become pregnant?

PROBLEM MANAGEMENT

Allergic reaction:
- Beware that latex powder can induce anaphylaxis and that the allergic reaction can precipitously increase in severity with continued exposure. Sometimes a person who ◄ says he (or she) is allergic to condoms may mean condoms are difficult to put on or lead to loss of erection or the couple simply doesn't like condoms. An ongoing infection may be attributed to condom "allergy"
- Switch to polyurethane condoms (Durex-Avanti, Trojan-Supra or Reality female condom) or stop using spermicide (depending on the suspected allergen)
- Some have suggested that a natural condom could be used as a sheath to protect the allergic member of the couple (placed beneath latex condom if man allergic or over the latex condom if woman allergic), but this could depend upon the severity of symptoms experienced
- Switch to another method, such as the female condom for STI risk reduction and a hormonal method for contraception

Condom breakage: (Figure 18.3, p. 54) (1-2% for latex condoms)
- Insure correct technique. Common problems: pre-placement manipulations (stretching, etc), use of inappropriate or incorrectly-placed lubricant, and prolonged or extremely vigorous sex
- May need to recommend larger condom
- If couple using polyurethane, consider switching to latex condom
- May need to switch method
- Confirm that woman is using ECPs and has supply available at home

Condom slippage: (Figure 18.3, p.54) (Slightly more common than condom breakage)
- Ensure correct technique. Common problems: condom not fully unrolled, lubricant placed incorrectly on inside of condom, and excessive delay in removing penis from vagina after ejaculation
- Rule out erectile dysfunction. Condoms may not be appropriate if man loses erection with condom placement or use
- Confirm that woman is using ECPs and has supply available at home

Decreased sensation:
- Common causes: condom too small, too thick or too tightly applied; inadequate lubrication
- Suggest experimentation with different textured condoms or placing second (larger size) condom over lubricated inner condom
- Integrate condom placement into lovemaking (suggest partner place condom to help arouse/excite man)

FERTILITY AFTER USE

- Immediate return to baseline fertility
- May protect fertility by reducing risk of cervical/urethral STIs, which can cause upper tract diseases and subsequent infertility

52

Figure 18.1

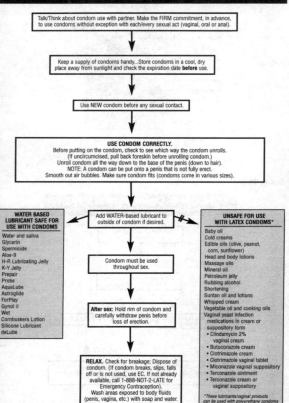

HOW TO USE A LATEX CONDOM
(...Or rubber, sheath, prophylactic, safe, french letter, raincoat, glove, sock)

Talk/Think about condom use with partner. Make the FIRM commitment, in advance, to use condoms without exception with each/every sexual act (vaginal, oral or anal).

Keep a supply of condoms handy...Store condoms in a cool, dry place away from sunlight and check the expiration date **before** use.

Use NEW condom before any sexual contact.

USE CONDOM CORRECTLY.
Before putting on the condom, check to see which way the condom unrolls.
(If uncircumcised, pull back foreskin before unrolling condom.)
Unroll condom all the way down to the base of the penis (down to hair).
NOTE: A condom can be put onto a penis that is not fully erect.
Smooth out air bubbles. Make sure condom fits (condoms come in various sizes).

WATER BASED LUBRICANT SAFE FOR USE WITH CONDOMS

Water and saliva
Glycerin
Spermicide
Aloe-9
H-R Lubricating Jelly
K-Y Jelly
Prepair
Probe
AquaLube
Astroglide
ForPlay
Gynol II
Wet
Cornhuskers Lotion
Silicone Lubricant
deLube

Add WATER-based lubricant to outside of condom if desired.

Condom must be used throughout sex.

After sex: Hold rim of condom and carefully withdraw penis before loss of erection.

RELAX. Check for breakage; Dispose of condom. (If condom breaks, slips, falls off or is not used, use EC. If not already available, call 1-888-NOT-2-LATE for Emergency Contraception.)
Wash areas exposed to body fluids (penis, vagina, etc.) with soap and water.

UNSAFE FOR USE WITH LATEX CONDOMS*

Baby oil
Cold creams
Edible oils (olive, peanut, corn, sunflower)
Head and body lotions
Massage oils
Mineral oil
Petroleum jelly
Rubbing alcohol
Shortening
Suntan oil and lotions
Vegetable oil and cooking oils
Whipped cream
Vaginal yeast infection medications in cream or suppository form
 • Clindamycin 2% vaginal cream
 • Butoconazole cream
 • Clotrimazole cream
 • Clotrimazole vaginal tablet
 • Miconazole vaginal suppository
 • Terconazole ointment
 • Terconazole cream or vaginal suppository

*These lubricants/vaginal products can be used with polyurethane condoms

53

Figure 18.2 Latex condom use and HIV infection in heterosexuals, 10 studies

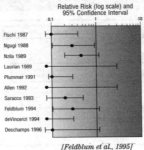

Relative Risk (log scale) and
95% Confidence Interval

Fischi 1987
Ngugi 1988
Nzila 1989
Laurian 1989
Plummer 1991
Allen 1992
Saracco 1993
Feldblum 1994
deVincenzi 1994
Deschamps 1996

[Feldblum et al., 1995]

Figure 18.3

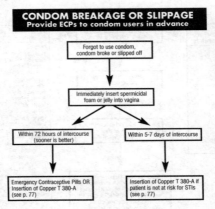

CONDOM BREAKAGE OR SLIPPAGE
Provide ECPs to condom users in advance

Forgot to use condom,
condom broke or slipped off

↓

Immediately insert spermicidal
foam or jelly into vagina

↓

Within 72 hours of intercourse
(sooner is better)

Within 5-7 days of intercourse

↓

Emergency Contraceptive Pills OR
Insertion of Copper T 380-A
(see p. 77)

Insertion of Copper T 380-A if
patient is not at risk for STIs
(see p. 77)

CHAPTER 19

Condoms for Women: Reality Female Condom
www.femalehealth.com ◄—

DESCRIPTION
A condom controlled by women. Considered by some to be condom that can empower women. Disposable, single-use polyurethane sheath, which is placed into the vagina. Flexible and movable inner ring at closed end is used to insert device into the vagina. Larger, fixed outer ring remains outside the vagina to cover part of introitus. Shelf life 3-5 years. When used as primary method, the female condom should be coupled with advance prescription of emergency contraceptive pills (ECPs)

EFFECTIVENESS [Trussell J. in Contraceptive Technology, 1998]
Perfect use failure rate in first year of use: 5% (Table 13.2, pg. 36)
Typical use failure rate in first year of use: 21%

MECHANISM
• The female condom acts as a mechanical barrier; it prevents pregnancy by preventing the passage of sperm into the female reproductive tract
• Sheathing the vagina and trapping the ejaculate also reduces transmission of bacterial and viral STIs

COST in 1995 [Trussell, 1995; Smith, 1993]

	Managed-Care Setting	Public Sector Setting
Published prices	$3.66	$1.25
Typical negotiated prices	$2.00-3.00	$0.70

ADVANTAGES
Menstrual: No impact on menses per se, but couple may feel more comfortable having ◄— intercourse during menses if a female condom is used
Sexual/psychology
• Intercourse may be more pleasurable because fear of pregnancy and STIs is decreased
• Can be inserted up to 8 hours before sex to allow more spontaneity
• If woman inserts it, she can be sure she is somewhat protected
• Makes sex less messy for the women after removal of the condom
Cancers/tumor, masses
• Possible decrease in HPV transmission may decrease risk of cervical dysplasia, cancer and genital warts (no data)
Other
• Available over-the-counter; no medical visit required
• Immediately active after placement
• Provides option to women whose partners can not or will not use male condom. May circumvent erectile concerns some men have with male condoms
• Reduces risk of STI transmission and acquisition, especially of cervical, vaginal infections and viral infections such as Hepatitis B. May decrease risk of HIV or HSV2. If used consistently and correctly, may reduce risk of PID and sequelae (infertility, ectopic pregnancy and chronic pelvic pain)
• Can be safely used by people with latex allergies or sensitivities

DISADVANTAGES

Menstrual: None

Sexual/psychology:

- Use may interrupt lovemaking unless woman places beforehand in anticipation of intercourse
- Requires careful sexual practices during intercourse (see INSTRUCTIONS FOR PATIENT), which may make intercourse awkward and less spontaneous
- May be difficult for woman to ask her partner to follow instructions for use
- Noise made during intercourse may be distracting (additional lubricant can quiet)

Cancers/tumors/masses: None

Other:

- Requires application with each act of intercourse (can be costly)
- Requires education and experience for successful use
- Somewhat difficult for new users (even experienced diaphragm users) to insert
- Couples may be embarrassed to purchase and to apply condoms due to taboos about touching genitalia

COMPLICATIONS

- Intravaginal methods can change vaginal flora and increase UTI risks

PRESCRIBING PRECAUTIONS

- Women unable to insert condom correctly and follow other instructions
- Women who require better pregnancy protection should at least combine the female condom and with a more effective method (not the male latex condom)
- Stress not to wash and reuse a second or third time unless having SI with same partner ◄

CANDIDATES FOR USE:

Virtually every woman qualifies medically to use the female condom. However, the female condom's relatively high cost, difficulty using it, and its high failure rate usually limit its use to women whose partners can not or will not use a male condom. Specific candidates include:

- Couples willing to accept relatively high failure rates
- Couples who need method directed by woman
- Women needing STI protection during pregnancy ◄
- Women needing protection postpartum (if intercourse not uncomfortable)

Special applications for infection control in couples not able to use male condoms:

- Non-monogamous couples (pregnant as well as if not pregnant)
- New couples
- After pregnancy or after pregnancy loss, to reduce risk of endometritis
- Couples with known chronic viral infections (HIV, HPV, HSV) involved in areas sheathed by device

Adolescents: May be offered method, but cost, problems with proper placement and high failure rate detract from its desirability

INITIATING METHOD

- Women planning to use the female condom need to have a chance to study instructions and practice inserting and using method prior to relying on it.
- Patients also benefit from counseling about:
  - How to negotiate with partner to be able to successfully use
  - Need to use with every act of intercourse
  - How to deal with device mishaps
- In addition, provide ECPs to women relying on female condoms for birth control to ensure immediate use after condom failures. This will minimize risk of unintended pregnancy

INSTRUCTIONS FOR PATIENT

- Each act of intercourse requires a new female condom
- Open packaging carefully. Avoid scissors or sharp objects that could cut or tear device
- Patient should rest comfortably in squat or lithotomy position
- Compress inner ring of device and introduce into vagina much like a diaphragm. Use inner ring to guide sheath high into vagina until the outer ring rests against vulva. Rotate inner ring to stabilize device in vault. Avoid tearing condom with jewelry. See package instructions for details and drawings illustrating insertion
- Penis must be manually placed (by either man or woman) into the sheath for intercourse
- Either woman or man should manually stabilize outer ring against perineum during intercourse to prevent loss of device into the vagina
- Man should monitor for any friction between penis and device which can cause condom breakage or device inversion
- Remove condom immediately after intercourse before arising. Test condom for patency and discard; the device can not be reused
- If there is any dislocation of the female condom during intercourse or any breakage or spillage of the ejaculate into genitalia, have patient place vaginal spermicide immediately and start her ECPs ASAP. If woman has no ECPs, have her call 1-888-NOT-2-LATE or check www.not-2-late.com/ to locate a provider of ECPs in her area. If at risk for STIs when condom fails, seek medical care.
- Never mix latex male condom and polyurethane female condom. The oil-based lubricant of the Reality female condom can cause breakage of latex male condoms. Friction between the condoms may cause breakage of either or both sheaths.

FOLLOW-UP

- Are you and your partner comfortable with your using the female condom?
- Have you had any problems using the female condom?
- Have you had intercourse—even once—without a female condom?
- Did you have any problem with ECPs? Do you need more ECPs?
- When do you plan to become pregnant?

PROBLEM MANAGEMENT

- Difficulty inserting device: Offer to formally (re)instruct patient.
- Problems with removal: Recommend relaxation techniques or have partner remove
- Condom dislodgement or inversion or penis inserted outside condom: Insert a new condom prior to continuing intercourse. Have patient take ECPs if any spill suspected. If at risk for STIs, seek medical care
- Recurrent UTIs with female condom use: Recommend precoital and postcoital urination. If not responsive, change method or offer antibiotic prophylaxis with intercourse

FERTILITY AFTER USE

- Immediate return to baseline fertility
- Female condom may protect fertility by reducing risk of cervical or vaginal STIs, which can cause upper tract disease and subsequent infertility

CHAPTER 20
Cervical Cap

DESCRIPTION

Prentif Cavity Rim Cervical Cap is a thimble-shaped latex rubber device with a small groove in its inner surface, which creates suction to keep cap on cervix. Four sizes are available with internal diameters of 22, 25, 28, 31 mm. A small amount of spermicide is placed inside the cap before it is placed over the cervix. When used as a primary method, cervical cap should be coupled with advance prescription of emergency contraceptive pills (ECPs)

EFFECTIVENESS (Rates include use with spermicide cream or jelly)

	Parous	Nulliparous
Perfect use failure rate in first year:	26%	9%
Typical use failure rate in first year:	40%	20%

[Trussell J in Contraceptive Technology, 1998] (See Table 13.2, p. 36)

MECHANISM

Acts both as a mechanical barrier to sperm migration into the cervical canal and as a chemical agent by applying the spermicide directly to the cervix

COST in 1995

	Managed-Care Setting	Public Provider Setting
Device	$31.00/3 years	$19.00/3 years
Office visit (device fitting)	38.00	15.59
Spermicidal jelly	12.00	8.75

[Trussell, 1995; Smith, 1993]

ADVANTAGES

Menstrual: None

Sexual/psychological
- Intercourse may be more pleasurable because fear of pregnancy and STIs is reduced
- Controlled by the woman
- Can be inserted up to 6 hours prior to sexual intercourse to permit spontaneity in love making
- Can remain in place for multiple acts of sexual intercourse for up to 48 hours

Cancers, tumors, and masses: None

Other:
- May reduce risk of cervical infections
- Immediately active after placement

DISADVANTAGES

Menstrual: None

Sexual/psychological
- Requires placement prior to genital contact, which may reduce spontaneity
- Some women do not like placing fingers or foreign body into vagina

Cancers, tumors, and masses
- Labeling requires repeat Pap smear at 3 months after initiation because increased risk of cervical dysplasia at 3 months; no increase at 1 year

Other:
- Lack of protection against some STIs and HIV. Must use condoms if at risk
- Relatively high failure rate, especially in parous women
- Requires professional fitting and requires formal (although brief) training
- About 80% of women can be fitted
- Severe obesity may make it difficult for patient to place correctly
- Odor may develop if cap left in place too long, if not appropriately cleansed, or if used during bacterial vaginosis

COMPLICATIONS
- UTIs may increase as vaginal flora changes to include higher coliform counts
- Cervical erosion may occur causing vaginal spotting and/or cervical discomfort. Some women change size of cervix during cycle and need two different size caps
- No cases of toxic shock have been reported, but theoretically, the risk may be increased, particularly if cap were left in for longer than recommended or used during menses
- Allergic reactions to latex may be life threatening; 2-3% of Americans (men and women) have a latex allergy; up to 14% of latex workers are sensitized

CANDIDATES FOR USE
- Women willing and able to insert device prior to coitus and remove it later
- Women with smooth cervix which can be fit successfully
- Women with pelvic relaxation are better candidates for cap than diaphragm
- Women and partner(s) who have no allergies to latex/spermicides

Adolescents: appropriate option, but fitting and insertion may be difficult and offers no protection against certain STIs including HIV

INITIATING METHOD
- The cervical cap must be professionally fit
- A speculum exam is required to judge the size and contour of the cervix, to evaluate for acute cervicitis and vaginitis, and to obtain a Pap smear
- If no nodules, lesions, cysts or other vaginal or cervical abnormalities preclude cap use, a rough estimate is made of the diameter of the cervix
- On bimanual exam, the uterine size and position, and the position, length and diameter of the cervix are determined
- Starting with the smallest likely size cap, squeeze the sides of the rim together and hold the cap with the dome pointing downward
- Apply a small amount of lubricant to the outside edge to facilitate insertion
- With the patient in the lithotomy position, separate her labia and gently insert the cap into the vagina. Guide it into place until the rim slides over the sides of the cervix
- Check for adequate cervical coverage, proper seal and position stability
- The dome of the cap should completely cover the cervix; the rim of the cap tucked snugly and evenly into the fornices; there should be no gap between rim and cervix
- The cap should adhere to the cervix firmly; it should not dislodge during the fitting exam
- To evaluate the fit, make a 360° sweep of the cap rim with the vaginal examining finger to search for gaps or exposed parts of the cervix
- If a gap is found, see if the rim can be pulled away with direct pressure
- After the cap has been in place for at least a minute, check the suction by pinching the excess rubber on the dome between the tips of two fingers and tugging
- The dome should dimple but should not collapse
- Cap should not be dislodged by manual manipulations such as gently pushing and tugging on it with one or two fingers from several angles

- After successful fitting, remove the cap by pushing the rim away from the cervix with one or two fingers to break the suction and then gently pull the cap out of the vagina
- Have patient demonstrate her ability to insert and remove cervical cap
- Provide ECPs in advance to enable immediate use after cervical cap dislodgement

INSTRUCTIONS FOR PATIENT TO USE

- Fill the bottom 1/3 of the inner aspect of the cap with 2% spermicide jelly and put the cap in place prior to sexual intercourse
- Test the fit to insure cervix is covered, with no gaps between the cervix and the cap; after suction develops for about 1 minute, check that the device does not dislodge with pressure
- Keep the cap in place for 6 hours after last sexual intercourse
- If multiple acts of sexual intercourse occur, there is no need to add more spermicide but do verify correct placement of the device before sexual intercourse
- Do not use the cap for more than 48 hours at a time, at the time of an infection, or during menses
- Do not expose the cap to petroleum-based products such as vaseline, baby oil, fungicidal creams and petroleum-based antibiotic creams (Listed in figure 18.1, p. 53)
- If cap dislodges, have patient start ECPs ASAP. If woman has no ECPs, have her call 1-888-NOT-2-LATE or check www.not-2-late.com to locate a provider of ECPs in her area.
- Use a backup method for first few uses until you are confident in your use of the cap
- Combining the cervical cap and the male condom can increase pregnancy protection
- The FDA recommends a follow-up Pap smear after 3 months
- Remove cap at least 2 or 3 days prior to Pap smears

HOW TO REMOVE

- Cap should not be removed until 6 hours after last ejaculation, but prior to 48 hours of use
- Insert a finger into the vagina until the rim of the cap is felt
- Press the cap rim until the seal against the cervix is broken; then tilt the cap off the cervix
- Hook finger around the rim and pull it sideways out of the vagina
- The device must be washed, rinsed, dried and stored in a cool, dark, and dry location. Rinsing in Listerine can prevent odors

FOLLOW-UP

_Are you or your partner experiencing any tenderness or irritation?
_Is the odor of the cap a problem?
_Do you use the cap every single time you have sexual intercourse?
_Do you have any problems with ECPs? Do you need more ECPs?
_When do you plan to become pregnant?

PROBLEM MANAGEMENT

- Allergic reaction to latex: Stop use and switch to another method
- Spotting/cervical tenderness/erosion: Stop use to allow healing; refit with larger cap; rule out STI
- Malodor of device: Listerine soaks may help; shorten time left in place, or replace cap
- Failure to use correctly: Use emergency contraception. If not already available, call 1-888-NOT-2-LATE or check www.not-2-late.com

FERTILITY AFTER USE: Immediate return to baseline fertility

DESCRIPTION

Rubber dome-shaped device filled with spermicide and placed to cover cervix; four types of diaphragms are available:

- Arcing spring: exerts pressure evenly around its rim to cover the cervix
- Coil spring: most appropriate for women with a deep pubic arch with average vaginal tone
- Flat spring: most appropriate with strong vaginal muscle tone or a shallow arch
- Wide seal: extends inward from the rim to contain the spermicide

EFFECTIVENESS (See Table 13.2, p. 36)

Perfect use failure rate in first year: 6%
Typical use failure rate in first year: 20%
[Trussell J in Contraceptive Technology, 1998]

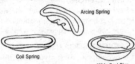

MECHANISM

Acts both as a mechanical barrier to sperm migration into the cervical canal and as a spermicide.

COST in 1995

	Managed-Care Setting	Public Provider Setting
Device	$18.00/3 yrs	$15.00/3 yrs
Office Visit (device fitting)	38.00	15.59
Spermicidal Jelly	12.00	8.75 *[Trussell, 1995; Smith, 1993]*

ADVANTAGES

Menstrual: None
Sexual/psychological:

- Controlled by the woman
- May be placed by the woman in anticipation of intercourse (within 6 hrs)
- May make sexual intercourse more enjoyable by reducing risk of pregnancy

Cancers, tumors, and masses: None
Other:

- Reduces risk for cervical STIs, including gonorrhea, chlamydia, cervical dysplasia, and PID
- Is used only with sexual intercourse
- May be used during lactation after vagina and cervix have achieved non-pregnant shape

DISADVANTAGES

Menstrual: None

Sexual/psychological:
- Requires placement prior to genital contact which can interrupt spontaneity of sexual intercourse
- Taste of spermicide may discourage certain foreplay activities
- May become messy with multiple acts of intercourse
- Some women dislike placing fingers or foreign bodies into vagina

Cancer, tumors, and masses: None

Other:
- Requires professional fitting; severe obesity may make fitting difficult
- May not be feasible for women with pelvic relaxation
- Requires brief, formal training in use and some dexterity to place and remove device
- May develop odor if not properly cleansed

COMPLICATIONS
- May increase risk of UTI, as result of increase in coliform count in vaginal flora
- May increase risk of TSS, especially if used for prolonged periods or during menses
- Large, poorly fitted diaphragm may cause vaginal erosions

CANDIDATES FOR USE
- Women who can predict when intercourse will occur
- Couples willing to interrupt sex to insert if not done beforehand ◄
- Highly motivated women willing to use with every coital act

Adolescents: Appropriate, if taught to use consistently and correctly; requires discipline

INITIATING METHOD
- Needs to be professionally fitted
- Examination with speculum will rule out any vaginal/cervical abnormalities
- On bimanual exam, introduce your third finger into the posterior fornix and tilt your wrist upward to mark where on your index finger/hand contacts the symphysis. Use that measurement as a guide to select the size diaphragm to use and place a fitting diaphragm in the vagina
- Check to ensure diaphragm is lodged behind symphysis and completely covers the cervix. Have patient bear down and visually check to ensure that diaphragm does not move from behind pubic arch
- Have woman walk around for a while in your office to test its long-term comfort
- Have woman demonstrate her ability to insert and remove diaphragm
- Encourage use of a backup method for first few uses to ensure correct use before relying exclusively on diaphragm for protection
- Suggest patient wear diaphragm for 6 hours before using it for contraception to ensure that it is comfortable and can be worn for 6 hours after intercourse
- Provide ECPs in advance!

INSTRUCTIONS FOR USE
- Fill inner surface of device 2/3's full with 2 teaspoons of spermicide prior to insertion. It can remain in place for up to 24 hours. Place in before genital contact but no longer than 6 hours before coitus

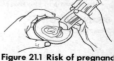

Figure 21.1 Risk of pregnanc increases when a spermicid is not used. Put spermicide on rim and on inside

- Prior to each act of coitus, reconfirm correct placement. For the second and each subsequent act, add additional spermicide vaginally but do not remove the device
- Leave in place for 6 hours after the last act of sexual intercourse
- Avoid using any petroleum-based vaginal products such as Vaseline, antifungal creams or some antibiotic creams. (See list of products UNSAFE to use with latex condoms on Figure 18.1, p. 53)
- After removal, clean with soap and water, rinse, dry, and store in the case in a cool, clean, dry, dark area
- Inspect periodically for any stiffness, holes, cracks, or other defects
- Have it checked each year by a professional. Replace at least every 2 years. Recheck for correct fit whenever there is a 20% weight change and after each pregnancy
- Combine diaphragm with male condoms to reduce pregnancy and STI risk
- If diaphragm dislodges or is not used properly, use EC

**Figure 21.2
Reconfirm correct placement of the diaphragm by feeling the cervix through the diaphragm**

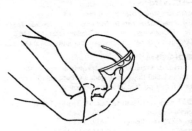

FOLLOW-UP

_Is the diaphragm comfortable? Do you feel excessive pressure?

_Do you get bladder infections often?

_Have you or your partner had an allergic reaction, i.e., burning or itching?

_Do you use the diaphragm consistently?

_Do you always apply a spermicide prior to insertion?

_Do you have any problems with ECPs? Do you need more ECPs?

_When do you plan to become pregnant?

PROBLEM MANAGEMENT

Prone to cystitis: Urinate postcoitally to reduce bladder colonization with vaginal bacteria

Allergy to latex: Discontinue use and discuss alternatives. Mylex makes a silicone diaphragm ◄—

FERTILITY AFTER USE: No adverse effects on fertility; may reduce risk of PID

DESCRIPTION

In the USA, nonoxynol-9 is available over the counter. In addition to N-9, patients around the world use menfegol, benzalkonium chloride, sodium docusate, and chlorhexidine. Spermicides are detergents that are available as vaginal creams, films, foams, gels, suppositories, sponges and tablets. When used as a primary method, spermicides should be coupled with advance prescription of emergency contraceptive pills (ECPs). The search for an ← effective vaginal microbicide that would also kill sperm remains an important research priority in reproductive health. Just under 50% of HIV infections world wide are now in women

EFFECTIVENESS (See Table 13.2, p. 36)

Perfect use failure rate in first year: 6%

Typical use failure rate in first year: 26%   *[Trussell J in Contraceptive Technology, 1998]*

• Note: recent study shows 6 month failure rates of 21-24%

• Combined with other methods, contraceptive and antimicrobial benefits increase

MECHANISM

As barriers, the vehicles prevent sperm from entering the cervical os. As detergents, the chemicals attack the sperm flagella and body, reducing mobility, and disrupting their fructolytic activity, jeopardizing nourishment

COST: Varies from state to state; 1995 national averages are:

Creams/Gels $10.08 for 8 oz

Film (VCF) (see figure) $12.26 for 12

Foam $11.23 for 0.6 oz

Suppositories/Tabs $12.79 for 18 inserts

ADVANTAGES

Menstrual: None

Sexual/psychological:

• Intercourse may be more pleasurable because fear of pregnancy is reduced

• Lubrication, in the case of foam, heightens satisfaction in both partners

• Ease in application (for some women) prior to sexual intercourse

• Either partner can purchase and apply; requires minimal negotiation

• May be used by woman without partner knowing

Cancers, tumors, and masses:

• Possible decrease in HPV transmission may reduce risk of cervical dysplasia and cancer

Other:

• May decrease risk of some vaginal and cervical STIs. Does not decrease risk of HIV

• Available over the counter; requires no medical visit

• Inexpensive for each individual use

• Easy to use

• Foam is immediately active with placement

DISADVANTAGES

Menstrual: None

Sexual/psychological

- Films and suppository spermicides require 10-15 minutes for activation, which may interrupt lovemaking
- Either partner must feel comfortable inserting fingers into vagina
- Insertion is not easy for some couples due to embarrassment or reluctance to touch genitalia
- Some forms, e.g., foam, become "messy" during intercourse
- Possible vaginal, oral, and anal irritation can disrupt or preclude sex
- Taste may be unpleasant

Cancers, tumors, and masses: None

Other:

- Not protective against transmission of HIV (see p. 140 - statement from CDC STI Treatment Guidelines); data are inconsistent as to whether N-9 prevents or increases transmission of HIV; may, in women having frequent intercourse with multiple partners, enhance transmission of HIV *[Van Dame, Durban, 2000 found 1.7 RR of HIV transmission in users of spermicidal vaginal gel with 52.5 mg N-9] [Kreiss - 1992]*
- Allergic reactions and dermatitis in women and men that could decrease compliance
- Might increase likelihood of STIs (including HIV) and UTIs by irritation of vaginal mucosa and by destroying vaginal flora, e.g., lactobacilli, in nonoxynol-9 concentrations as low as 0.1%

COMPLICATIONS

- Women and men have confused fruit jelly, e.g., grape jelly, for spermicidal "jelly"
- Women and men have attempted to use cosmetics or hair products containing non-spermicidal octoxynols and nonoxynols (nonoxynol 4, 10, 12, and 14) in lieu of nonoxynol-9

CANDIDATES FOR USE

- Any woman who presents with no prior allergy or reaction to spermicides

Adolescents:

- Readily available and not contraindicated for teens
- High failure rate may discourage long-term use as primary method

INITIATING METHOD

- Except in cases where the patient, or partner, presents with pregnancy, allergy, or irritation, women can begin these methods at any time following product instructions
- Provide ECPs in advance

INSTRUCTIONS FOR PATIENT

- Before and after applying spermicide, inserting person should wash and dry hands
- Spermicide container must have active date and no defects
- Spermicide has its greatest efficacy near the cervical os
- Encourage more spermicide for each act of sexual intercourse
- Water exposure, e.g. bathing or douching, within 6 hours after insertion or post-coitally can minimize effectiveness; reapply before next penetrative act
- Keep spermicides in cool, dry places; tablets or foam can tolerate heat, film melts at 98.6° F

Creams/foams/gels
- Apply less than 1 hour prior to sexual intercourse. May drip out of vagina if inserted more than 1 hour in advance. With foam, shake canister vigorously. Fill plastic applicator with spermicide. Insert applicator deeply into vagina and depress plunger. Immediately active. Finish sexual intercourse within 60 minutes of application

Film, suppositories and tablets
- Insert at least 15 minutes before sexual intercourse: with film, fold the sheet in half and then half again (this aids insertion). Using fingers or an applicator, the inserting partner places the spermicide applicator or film deeply in the vagina, hopefully near cervix. Finish sexual intercourse within 60 minutes of application

FOLLOW-UP

_Have you or your partner(s) experienced any rash or discomfort after using spermicides?
_Have you changed partners since beginning spermicides?
_Have you had sex—even once—without using spermicides?
_Did you have problems with ECPs?
_Do you need more ECPs?
_When do you plan to become pregnant?

PROBLEM MANAGEMENT

Dermatitis: Discontinue spermicides and offer another method. If vehicle served as lubricant, recommend a water-based or silicone-based lubricant without nonoxynol-9 or octoxynol-9

Changed partners: Explain STI prevention and check for STIs

FERTILITY AFTER USE: Immediate return to baseline fertility

LATE BREAKING NEWS: For thousands of years, women have placed sponges with a variety of spermicides into the vagina. As this book was going to press, we learned that the Today Contraceptive Sponge is likely to be back on US pharmacy shelves by the end of 2001. The newer low estimates of spermicidal effectiveness need to be discussed with interested women. Clinicians may be able to help women learn how to insert and remove the sponge. Call (201) 934-4449 for further information, to order Today Sponges, and to request educational materials.

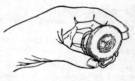

DESCRIPTION
Man withdraws penis completely from the vagina before ejaculation

EFFECTIVENESS
Perfect use failure rate in first year: 4% (See Table 13.2, p. 36)
Typical use failure rate in first year: 19%
[Trussell J in Contraceptive Technology, 1998]

MECHANISM
Withdrawal prior to ejaculation reduces or eliminates sperm introduced into vagina.
Preejaculatory fluid is not generally a problem unless two acts of sexual intercourse are
close together.

COST: None

ADVANTAGES
Menstrual: None
Sexual/psychological:
- No barriers
- Readily available method which encourages male involvement
- May introduce variety into sexual relationship

Cancers, tumors, and masses: None
Other: Surprisingly effective if used correctly

DISADVANTAGES
Menstrual: None
Sexual/psychological
- May not be applicable for couples with sexual dysfunction such as premature ejaculation
  or unpredictable ejaculation
- Requires man's cooperation and instruction
- May reduce sexual pleasure of woman and intensity of orgasm of man
- Encourages "spectatoring" or thinking about what is happening during sexual intercourse

Cancers, tumors, and masses: None
Other: Relatively high failure rate among typical users and does not protect against STIs

COMPLICATIONS: None

MEDICAL ELIGIBILITY CHECKLIST
- Man must be able to predict ejaculation in time to withdraw penis completely from vagina
  and introitus
- Premature ejaculation makes method less effective
- Appropriate for couples not at risk for STIs

CANDIDATES FOR USE

- Couples who are able to communicate during sexual intercourse
- Disciplined men who can ignore the powerful instinct, urging them to continue thrusting
- Couples in stable, mutually monogamous relationship
- Couples without religious or cultural prohibitions against withdrawal
- Women willing to accept higher risk of unintended pregnancy

Adolescents: Compliance may be a problem (as it is for couples of all ages); teens may have less control over ejaculation; advise use of condoms for better protection against pregnancy and STIs. While withdrawal is a relatively poor contraceptive option, especially if ◄—— pregnancy prevention and infection control are very important, withdrawal is definitely better than using no contraceptive at all

INITIATING METHOD: Can begin at any time; provide ECPs in advance

INSTRUCTIONS FOR PATIENT

- Practice withdrawal using backup method until both partners master withdrawal
- Wipe penis clean of the pre-ejaculation fluid prior to vaginal penetration
- Use coital positions that reduce deep vaginal penetration: 1) male partial penetration in the male superior position, 2) the female superior position, and 3) side-by-side or spooning
- Use emergency contraception if withdrawal fails

FOLLOW-UP

_Do your partner(s) ever ejaculate/begin to ejaculate before withdrawing?
_Did you have any problems with ECPs? Do you need more ECPs?
_When do you want to become pregnant?

PROBLEM MANAGEMENT

Failure to withdraw: Use ECPs if withdrawal does not occur every time

FERTILITY AFTER USE: No adverse effects on fertility

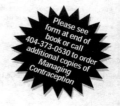

Please see form at end of book or call 404-373-0530 to order additional copies of Managing Contraception

CHAPTER 24

Emergency Contraception

www.not-2-late.com or www.opr.princeton.edu/ec

OVERVIEW

Emergency contraception (EC) includes any method that acts after intercourse to *prevent pregnancy*. There are currently 3 methods in widespread use worldwide:

- Yuzpe Method with combined oral contraceptive pills (COCs)
- High-dose progestin-only contraceptive pills (POPs)
- Copper IUD insertion

A poll of pre-med students at Stanford found that not one knew that some already existing birth control pills are options for emergency contraception. *"Amazing but true,"* noted Martha Campbell Ph.D. *[personal communication-1/1/01]* In much of the world including many U.S. pharmacies, dedicated products to prevent pregnancy after unprotected sex are not available. Campbell and her husband Dr. Malcolm Potts raise this important question: *"How many unwanted pregnancies could we be averting if we could tell everyone what's possible with what they already have on hand?"*

Only the two hormonal methods using emergency contraceptive pills (ECPs) are utilized to any significant degree in the U.S. (all combined and progestin-only pills that may be used are on p. 74 of this book and in colored diagram on p. 87). None of the current methods is an abortifacient; none disturbs an implanted pregnancy. Both hormonal methods are more effective the *sooner* they are started after intercourse. Provide to patients in advance in one of 2 ways: give them pills in advance or give them a prescription in advance (a prescription with refills!)

Table 24.1 Overview of Postcoital Methods Currently Available in U.S.

Characteristic	COCs	POPs	Copper IUD
Timing of initiation after intercourse	**Can** be used after 72 hours; Sooner is better	**Can** be used after 72 hours; Sooner is better	Up to 5-7 days
Pregnancies/ 100 women	Early start: 0.5% Late start: 4.2% Average: 2 - 3.2%	Early start: 0.4% Late start: 2.7% Average: 1.1%	0.1%
Advantages	Product available for advance prescription: PREVEN™; Wide range of COCs available for use	Fewer side effects than EC with COCs; Product available for advance prescription: Plan B®	May be inserted 5 or more days after intercourse, but before implantation. Effective long-term contraceptive for appropriate women
Disadvantages	Gastrointestinal side effects – can be reduced with antiemetic pretreatment	Plan B currently has somewhat limited availability; can use Ovrette (20 pills each dose) in interim	Expensive; must be appropriate candidate for IUD; Timing issues: counseling, testing, etc. Insertion procedure required
Side effects	Nausea, vomiting, headache, breast tenderness, moodiness, change in next menses	Same hormonal side effects as COCs, but less frequent and less severe	Pain, bleeding, expulsion
Avoid use in pregnant women and women with other prescribing precautions	Avoid use in women with known pregnancy or current severe migraine. POPs a better option for women with migraine	Avoid use in women with known pregnancy; the treatment will not be effective	Prescribing precautions for IUD use (see page 80)

For more information about EC, phone numbers of EC providers, or to become listed as an EC provider, check out the internet web site at www.not-2-late.com or call the EC Hotline at 1-888-NOT-2-LATE. Other good sources of information about EC are www.preven.com or 1-888-PREVEN-2 and www.go2planB.com or call 800-330-1271.

DESCRIPTION

POPs:
- Two doses of progestin (0.75 mg of levonorgestrel or 1.5 mg of norgestrel in each dose). Take first dose as soon as possible within 72 hours after unprotected or inadequately protected sexual intercourse; take second dose 12 hours later (second dose may be more than 72 hours after unprotected sex)
- Plan B is the only currently-available FDA-approved progestin-only product with instructions and pills that facilitate advance prescription
- Ovrette (20 yellow pills for each dose; she needs 2 packs of Ovrette)

Yuzpe Method using COCs:
- Two large doses of COCs with at least 100 µg of ethinyl estradiol and either 100 mg of norgestrel or 50 mg of levonorgestrel. Take first dose as soon as possible within 72 hours after unprotected or inadequately protected sexual intercourse; take second dose 12 hours later (second dose may be more than 72 hours after unprotected sex) Try to provide ECPs to women in advance (either actual pills or prescription with refills).
- The PREVEN™ Emergency Contraceptive Kit is the only currently available FDA-approved product that facilitates utilizing combined OCs advance prescription with instructions for and pills for each dose
- Other COCs with appropriate progestins may be prescribed (see Figure 24.1, p. 76)

EFFECTIVENESS

EC with POPs PLAN B	Only 1.1% of 967 women using POPs for EC became pregnant in a WHO multi-center study *[WHO task force on Postovulatory Methods of Fertility Regulation. Lancet Aug 8, 1998]*	85% average reduction of pregnancy rate	12 pregnancies per 1000 unprotected acts of sexual intercourse followed by EC
EC with COCs Preven	2-3% failure rate	60-75% average reduction of pregnancy rate	20-32 pregnancies per 1000 unprotected acts of sexual inter-course followed by EC

- In WHO study effectiveness was greater the sooner ECPs are taken. Only 4 pregnancies per 1000 unprotected acts of sexual intercourse if ECPs taken within the first 12 hours (95% reduction in pregnancy rate)
- Soon to be published study demonstrates that ECPs remain effective for 5 days after unprotected sex
- Taking more than number of pills specified is not beneficial and may increase risk of vomiting

MECHANISMS

- ECPs act primarily as contraceptives, sometimes as interceptives, and never as abortifacients
- If taken before ovulation, ECPs disrupt normal follicular development and maturation, block LH surge, and inhibit ovulation; they may also create deficient luteal phase
- If taken after ovulation, ECPs have little effect on ovarian hormonal production and limited effect on endometrial maturation
- ECPs may affect tubal transport of sperm or ova

COST

POPs:
- Plan B is not available in all retail pharmacies as of December 2000, but distribution is improving. Plan B has been sold in family planning clinics for less than $5 per cycle
- Ovrette (2 packs) is not readily available in all pharmacies and can cost up to $60

Yuzpe method with COCs:
- The PREVEN™ kit: Pills plus pregnancy test: $20-$25 at retail pharmacies. Publicly supported clinics can buy PREVEN™ kit less expensively.
- One cycle of COCs may vary from a few dollars to more than $50. Ovral tends to be more expensive than other combined pills and is not carried in all drug stores.

Other costs:
- Cost prior to obtaining pills may vary from nothing (if given) to the cost of a phone call to the cost of a full exam and pregnancy test.

ADVANTAGES

Menstrual: None

Sexual/Psychological:
- Offers an opportunity to prevent pregnancy after rape, mistake, or overt barrier method failure (condom breaks or slips, diaphragm dislodges, etc.)
- Reduces anxiety about unintended pregnancy prior to next menses
- Process of getting EC may lead woman to initiate ongoing contraception

Cancers, tumors and masses: None

Other:
- Reduces ectopic pregnancy rate
- There are 3 million unintended pregnancies each year; nearly half of all pregnancies are unintended, and half of all women aged 15-44 have had an unintended pregnancy *[Henshaw, 1998]* Widespread availability of ECPs could halve the number of unintended pregnancies and the consequent need for abortion *[Trussell, 1992]*
- Could also reduce birth defects (poor use of folic acid if conception is not planned) ◄—

DISADVANTAGES

Menstrual:
- Next menses may be early (especially if taken before ovulation), on time, or late
- Notable changes in menstrual flow seen in 10-15% of women

Sexual/psychological:
- Women who are uncomfortable with post-fertilization methods might need reassurance that use of EC with COCs or POPs is consistent with their beliefs if taken during the follicular phase. They also may need to be warned that if taken after ovulation, ECPs may work as an interceptive (ie prevent implantation of fertilized egg)

Cancers, tumors and masses: None

Other:
- Breast tenderness, fatigue, headache, abdominal pain and dizziness
- No protection against STIs; consider treatment for possible STIs following exposure

Nausea and vomiting:

	Nausea	Vomiting	Pretreatment with antiemetic
POPs	23%	6%	Helpful, but needed less often
COCs	50%	19%	Can reduce symptoms by 30-50% (see INITIATING METHOD, p. 72)

COMPLICATIONS
- Several cases of DVT reported in women using COCs as ECPs; probably not an attributable risk. No DVT risk with POPs

CANDIDATES FOR USE

• All women who have had or who may be at risk for unprotected sexual intercourse (sperm exposure) are candidates for ECPs for immediate or future use, but women with strong contraindications to estrogen use should use POPs not COCs as ECPs (see PRESCRIBING PRECAUTIONS)
• There are many situations in which women have unintended sperm exposure:
  • Failed contraceptive methods: broken condom, dislodged diaphragm, or cervical cap, forgotten pills, late for contraceptive reinjection, NFP miscalculation, failed withdrawal
  • Failure to use methods: clouded judgment, passion, sexual assault
• Note: ECPs do not protect as well as other ongoing methods, so there are few situations in which they would be offered as first-line protection

Adolescents: appropriate back-up option (consider providing ECPs in advance)

PRESCRIBING PRECAUTIONS

Labeling for Plan B (and therefore, by extension, for all POPs used for EC) lists only 3 prescribing precautions:
• Pregnancy
• Hypersensitivity to any component of product
• Undiagnosed abnormal vaginal bleeding

It might also be prudent to only use EC with POPs for women who breast-feed

Labeling for the PREVEN kit (and therefore, by extension, for all COCs used for EC) lists a wide range of contraindications. This list was inherited from the labeling for COCs used on an ongoing basis. In reality, use of COCs should be allowed for all women except those who:
• Are pregnant (no benefit)
• Are known to be hypersensitive to any component of the product
• Have acute migraine headaches at the time ECPs are to be taken
• Have history of DVT or PE (use POPs - PLAN B or Ovrette)

INITIATING METHOD: pregnancy testing optional, not required

• Offer ECPs routinely to all women who may be at risk for unprotected intercourse
  • Advance prescription increases use of EC but does not diminish use of primary method of contraception
  • Availability directly through pharmacists led to a thousand-fold increase in use of ECPs in selected pharmacies in the state of Washington
  • Self-contained kits such as PREVEN and Plan B, which come with FDA-approved instructions, are best for this "ECs to go"
• Provide EC for all women who present after-the-fact, acutely in need. If you dispense the pills in your clinic, have her remove the inactive pills to reduce risk of mistake.
• Elements needed from patient history:
  • LMP, previous menstrual period, dates of any prior unprotected intercourse this cycle, and date and time of last unprotected intercourse
  • Any problems with previous use of ECPs, COCs or POPs?
  • Breast-feeding or severe headaches now? History of DVT or PE? (Use POPs rather than COCs)
  • Any foreseeable problems if antiemetic causes drowsiness?
• No physical exam/labs needed on a routine basis:
  • No pelvic exam is necessary, now or in the past
  • No BP measurements needed in asymptomatic women
  • Pregnancy testing useful only if concerned that prior intercourse may have caused pregnancy. *ACOG, IPPF and WHO do not include routine pregnancy testing in their protocols*
• Advise patient about possible side effects and consider other EC options (Copper IUD)

72

- Premedicate with long-acting antiemetic one hour prior to first ECP dose if possible to minimize GI side effects. Take two tablets of meclizine hydrochloride 25 mg (over-the-counter Dramamine II or Bonine). Other agents work, but do not have same duration of action. Avoid this medication if drowsiness will pose safety hazard or inconvenience
- Offer appropriate number of tablets for particular ECP brand to reach adequate dose (see Figure 24.1, p.76 and p. A-22)
- Encourage patient to take second dose approximately 12 hours after first dose. Mid-afternoon first dose requires middle-of-the-night awakening for the second dose. Need to have patient help balance between need to take ECPs as soon as possible (for better efficacy) and need to ensure that second dose is taken (also needed for efficacy)
- Realize that 72 hours is not the absolute limit, particularly if patient is still early (follicular phase) in cycle so ECPs could still block ovulation
- Consider providing EC kit now for patient to have available at home in case she has another need to use EC again OR provide prescription with refills

STARTING REGULAR USE OF CONTRACEPTIVE AFTER USE OF ECPs
- Start using method immediately. There is no lingering reliable protection provided by ECPs
- If missed OCs, restart day after ECPs taken (no need to catch up missed pills)
- If starting OCs:
  - May wait for next menses or
  - Start OCs next day with 7-day backup method (this will affect timing of next menses)
- If starting DMPA injections, can start immediately. If so, consider having patient return in 2-3 weeks for pregnancy test
- If starting barrier methods, start immediately.
- If starting NFP, use abstinence (or barrier/spermicide) until next menses (date of ovulation and mucus production will be changed by ECPs)

SPECIAL ISSUES/FREQUENT QUESTIONS
- When in cycle should EC be offered? Anytime except perhaps if she is having her menses
- How many times a year can a woman use ECPs? No limit except that it would be better to have the patient use an ongoing preventive contraceptive because ECPs are less effective and more expensive than other methods. Third party payers may set maximum number of reimbursable uses per year
- What if a patient has had unprotected intercourse earlier in the cycle? Do urine test to confirm no obvious pregnancy. Offer EC. Advise that EC will not work if she already has (undetectable) pregnancy, but that it will not adversely affect the fetus or the pregnancy
- What if she used EC earlier in the month? Offer it again; she may have just delayed ovulation. Review why her primary contraceptive is failing her and remedy the situation (perhaps with a new method). Consider performing pregnancy test in this setting even though it may be too early to have meaning
- What happens if I do not offer EC? The courts have been very clear in their decisions that EC is standard of care and a provider faces liability for wrongful life if s/he does not offer EC (at least by referral)
- What if the pharmacy is closed or does not carry EC? Plan ahead—provide EC by advance prescription. Or offer EC using conventional COCs or POPs
- What if a woman whom I have not seen previously calls for ECPs? What can I do to help her? Many practitioners screen over the telephone and telephone in prescriptions to pharmacies. Documentation and billing are the only real issues, not medical appropriateness. If you register as an EC provider by phone or by internet, you will need to be prepared to address this issue.

INSTRUCTIONS FOR PATIENT

- For advance prescriptions, advise woman who is using COCs to purchase long-lasting antiemetic and keep it next to ECPs
- Make sure woman using antiemetic with COCs understands risk of drowsiness. Have her take antiemetic as soon as possible after unprotected sexual intercourse. Wait no longer than an hour to take first dose of ECPs
- Wait 12 hours, then take second dose of ECPs (Second dose of antiemetic unnecessary if long-acting antiemetic was used)
- Start using protection right away. ECPs do not reliably protect you beyond the day they are used
- Return for pregnancy testing if she has not had her menses 21 days after using ECPs
- Re-evaluate primary method to make it more reliable

FOLLOW-UP

- No routine follow-up needed
- Have patient return for pregnancy testing if no menses in 3 weeks

PROBLEM MANAGEMENT

Nausea/vomiting:

- In general, POPs are preferable because they are more effective and have lower risk of complications and side effects
- Antiemetic may be prescribed before or after taking combined COCs as ECPs (does not work as well when taken late)
- Vomiting that occurs due to ECPs probably indicates that enough hormones reached the bloodstream to have the desired contraceptive effect. Most experts (but NOT all) recommend a repeat dose of ECPs if vomiting occurs within 30 minutes of taking ECPs. ACOG recommends a repeat dose if vomiting occurs within one hour *[ACOG 1996]*
- If repeating dose because of severe vomiting, switch from COCs to POPs or consider placing pills in vagina rather than mouth (off-label). Although uptake is slower, this may also be possible for woman who has experienced extreme nausea while taking COCs in the past as her regular contraceptive

Amenorrhea:

- If menses do not occur in 21 days (or more than 7 days beyond expected day for menses to begin), need to rule out pregnancy

Pregnancy in spite of using ECPs:

- If there is a pregnancy, the woman should be reassured that there is no evidence in 25 years of use that ECPs increase the risk of fetal anomalies or disruption of pregnancy

FERTILITY AFTER USE

Excellent. Fertility returns after next menses (maybe before!)

EMERGENCY CONTRACEPTION WITH COPPER IUD

DESCRIPTION

- Insert Copper IUD, following the usual procedures, within 5 days after unprotected or inadequately protected sexual intercourse. May be used up to 8 days after intercourse, if ovulation is known to have occurred 3 days or more after the unprotected sex
- More frequently used overseas, where IUD costs are lower and IUD candidate restrictions are less stringent
- In the US, this method is generally restricted to use by women who intend to continue to use the IUD as an ongoing method; the choice should be the patient's

EFFECTIVENESS
- Failure rate < 1% (only about 6 pregnancies per 1000 insertions in world's literature)

MECHANISMS
- Usually functions as interceptive (after fertilization, but prior to implantation) by interfering with implantation
- Rarely, may act as contraceptive, if inserted days before ovulation

COST
- Extremely expensive unless used as a long-term contraceptive method after insertion as EC (see Chapter 25, p. 78-84). In Europe postcoital IUD insertion costs just $25 (Belgium) ◄ or is covered by health plan

ADVANTAGES
- The most effective post-coital method
- May be used two days later than ECPs
- Provides long-term protection against pregnancy following insertion

DISADVANTAGES: Same as using Copper IUD as contraceptive (See Chapter 25, p. 78-84)
- Very expensive, if only used for EC and removal expected soon
- Timing constraints of EC use may make it difficult to properly screen patients for IUD insertion (counseling, preinsertion cultures, etc.)

COMPLICATIONS, CANDIDATES FOR USE, PRESCRIBING PRECAUTIONS, INITIATING METHOD, INSTRUCTIONS FOR PATIENT FOLLOW-UP, PROBLEM MANAGEMENT, FERTILITY AFTER USE
- Same as using Copper IUD as ongoing contraceptive (See Chapter 25, p. 78-84)

EMERGENCY CONTRACEPTION WITH MIFEPRISTONE (RU-486)

DESCRIPTION
- Single 10 mg dose of the anti-progestogen mifepristone (RU-486), taken within 5 days of unprotected intercourse. Not available in the United States

EFFECTIVENESS
- Prevented over 98% of pregnancies
- One international study allowed initiation up to 120 hours and still found 85% overall efficacy

MECHANISMS
- Blocks action of progesterone by binding to its receptors
- Stops ovulation if given in follicular phase (contraceptive)
- Slows endometrial maturation in luteal phase (interceptive)

FERTILITY AFTER USE
- Fertility may return later in cycle or with next menses

Figure 24.1

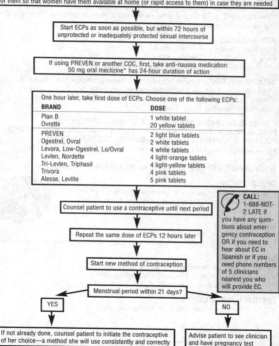

EMERGENCY CONTRACEPTION USING EMERGENCY CONTRACEPTIVE PILLS (ECPs)
Call 1-888-NOT-2 LATE; www.opr.princeton.edu/ec

Consider dispensing emergency contraceptive pills (ECPs) (or a prescription for ECPs) **prior to the need** for them so that women have them available at home (or rapid access to them) in case they are needed

Start ECPs as soon as possible, but within 72 hours of unprotected or inadequately protected sexual intercourse

If using PREVEN or another COC, first, take anti-nausea medication: 50 mg oral meclizine* has 24-hour duration of action

One hour later, take first dose of ECPs. Choose one of the following ECPs:

BRAND	DOSE
Plan B	1 white tablet
Ovrette	20 yellow tablets
PREVEN	2 light blue tablets
Ogestrel, Ovral	2 white tablets
Levora, Low-Ogestrel, Lo/Ovral	4 white tablets
Levlen, Nordette	4 light-orange tablets
Tri-Levlen, Triphasil	4 light-yellow tablets
Trivora	4 pink tablets
Alesse, Levlite	5 pink tablets

Counsel patient to use a contraceptive until next period

Repeat the same dose of ECPs 12 hours later

Start new method of contraception

Menstrual period within 21 days?

YES

NO

If not already done, counsel patient to initiate the contraceptive of her choice—a method she will use consistently and correctly

Advise patient to see clinician and have pregnancy test

CALL: 1-888-NOT-2 LATE if you have any questions about emergency contraception OR if you need to hear about EC in Spanish or if you need phone numbers of 5 clinicians nearest you who will provide EC.

NOTE: if anti-nausea medication is NOT taken prior to first dose of ECPs (which is recommended), it may be taken after the first dose, should nausea be severe or should woman vomit. Anti-nausea medication is usually not needed for women using PLAN B, as PLAN B does not contain estrogen.

76 * Meclizine hydrochloride is recommended because it has a 24-hour duration of action. It is available over the counter as Bonine and as Dramamine 2. If prescribing an antiemetic, use Antivert®. Other medications to prevent nausea may be prescribed instead.

Figure 24.2

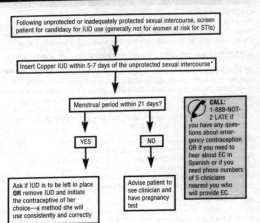

EMERGENCY CONTRACEPTION USING COPPER IUD
www.opr.princeton.edu/ec ◄

Following unprotected or inadequately protected sexual intercourse, screen patient for candidacy for IUD use (generally not for women at risk for STIs)

Insert Copper IUD within 5-7 days of the unprotected sexual intercourse*

Menstrual period within 21 days?

YES

NO

Ask if IUD is to be left in place **OR** remove IUD and initiate the contraceptive of her choice—a method she will use consistently and correctly

Advise patient to see clinician and have pregnancy test

CALL:
1-888-NOT-2 LATE if you have any questions about emergency contraception OR if you need to hear about EC in Spanish or if you need phone numbers of 5 clinicians nearest you who will provide EC.

* The Copper IUD may be inserted up to the time of implantation—about 5 days after ovulation—to prevent pregnancy. Thus, if a woman had unprotected sexual intercourse 3 days before ovulation occurred in that cycle, the IUD could be inserted up to 8 days after intercourse to prevent pregnancy

CHAPTER 25
Intrauterine Contraceptives
www.popcouncil.org, www.avsc.org, www.berlex.com,
www.paragardIUD.com, www.arhp.org ←

OVERVIEW

Three intrauterine contraceptives are currently available in the U.S.: the ParaGard® T 380A Intrauterine Copper (Copper IUD), the Progestasert® System progesterone-releasing contraceptive and the Mirena® levonorgestrel-releasing intrauterine system.

INTRAUTERINE COPPER CONTRACEPTIVE (ParaGard T 380A)

DESCRIPTION

T-shaped intrauterine contraceptive made of radiopaque polyethylene, with two flexible arms that bend for insertion but open in situ to hold solid sleeves of copper against fundus. Fine copper wire wrapped around stem. Surface area of copper = 380 mm². Monofilament polyethylene tail string threaded through and knotted below blunt ball at base of stem creates double strings that protrude into vagina. For medical information: 1-800-682-6532

EFFECTIVENESS *(Trussell J in Contraceptive Technology, 1998)*

• Approved for 10 years use; effective for at least 12 years.

Perfect use failure rate in first year: 0.6% (see Table 13.2, p. 36)
Typical use failure rate in first year: 0.8%
Cumulative 10-year failure rate: 2.1-2.8%

• Failure rates slightly higher in nulliparous women.

MECHANISMS

The intrauterine copper contraceptive works as a functional spermicide. Copper ions inhibit sperm motility and acrosomal enzyme activation so that sperm rarely reach the tube and are unable to fertilize the ovum. The inflammatory reaction created in the endometrium phagocytizes the sperm. There is no experimental evidence suggesting that the IUDs routinely work after fertilization. There is clear evidence that they are not abortifacients. They prevent pregnancy by preventing fertilization

COST in 1995

Setting:	Managed Care	Public Sector
Device	$184	109
Insertion (including screening, testing, counseling)	207	64
Uncomplicated removal (Trussell, 1995; Smith, 1993)	70	11

Special Cost Savings Programs: For full-pay purchasers of this IUD: 1-800-322-4966

• 3-month warranty. Manufacturer offers to replace any unit that is lost or must be removed within the first 3 months of use.

• Professional courtesy program: any staff member or relative of provider is eligible for a free unit.

• Manufacturer offers free IUD to patients experiencing financial problems who would otherwise not be able to afford a unit if the provider will insert the IUD free of charge. Forms are available from Ortho-McNeil representative

78

ADVANTAGES

Menstrual: none

Sexual/psychological
- Convenient; permits spontaneous sexual activities. Requires no action at time of use
- Intercourse may be more pleasurable with risk of pregnancy reduced

Cancers, tumors and masses
- Possible protection against endometrial and cervical cancer (case control studies)

Other
- Rapid return to fertility
- Convenient - single insertion and monthly string checks provide up to 12 years protection
- Private: partner usually not able to detect if properly placed
- Cost effective. Provides greatest net benefits of any contraceptive over a 5 year period. Every copper IUD inserted saves the health care system $14,133 in its first 5 years of use
- Good option for women who cannot use hormonal method
- Decreased risk for ectopic pregnancy
- IUDs lead to highest level of patient satisfaction of any contraceptive ⬅

DISADVANTAGES

Menstrual
- Average monthly blood loss increased by about 35%
- May increase dysmenorrhea (removal rates for bleeding and pain first year = 11.9%)
- Spotting and cramping with insertion and intermittently in weeks following insertion

Sexual/psychological
- Some women uncomfortable with concept of having "something" (foreign body) placed inside them
- Some women are not at ease checking string
- Strings palpable; if strings cut too short, may cause partner discomfort

Cancers, tumors and masses: None.

Other
- Requires office procedure for insertion and removal, which may be uncomfortable.
- Increases risk of infection in first 20 days after insertion (1/1000 women will get PID).
- Offers no protection from HIV/STIs; PID: see data in box below
- May be expelled obviously (with cramping and bleeding) or silently (placing unknowing woman at risk for pregnancy). Rate of expulsion declines over time. At 5 years ⬅ cumulative explusion rate is 11.3%. Expulsion rate for the 5th year is 0.3%

COMPLICATIONS

- See PROBLEM MANAGEMENT section for details

Complication	Frequency	Risk factors
PID within 20 days	1/1000	BV, cervicitis, contamination with insertion
Uterine perforation	1/1000	Immobile, markedly verted uterus Breast-feeding woman Inexperienced, unskilled inserter
Vasovagal reaction or Fainting with insertion	Rare	Stenotic os, pain Prior vasovagal reaction
Expulsion		Insertion on menses, too soon postpartum, or not high enough in fundus
Pregnancy		None known

CANDIDATES FOR USE

➤ • Women wanting long-term contraception but wanting to avoid tubal sterilization
• Recommended patient profile includes parous women in stable mutually monogamous relationships (at low risk of STIs) with no history of PID. The copper IUD and LNG IUD are best for women seeking longer-term (≥ 2 years) pregnancy protection due to its initial cost. However, nulliparous women at low risk for STIs may also be candidates. Women with history of PID may be candidates if they are currently in stable mutually monogamous relationships and have had a pregnancy since the PID episode
• Good option for women who cannot use hormones:
  • Women with personal risk of thrombosis
  • Breast-feeding women
  • Smokers over 35
  • Women who fear hormonal side effects

Adolescents: Only a few adolescents meet all the criteria for IUD use.

PRESCRIPTION PRECAUTIONS:

• Pregnancy
• Women at risk for STIs (multiple sex partners)
• Uterus < 6 cm or > 9 cm
• Undiagnosed abnormal vaginal bleeding
• Cervicitis or pelvic infection or actinomycosis
• Recent endometritis (last 3 months)
• Allergy to copper; Wilson's disease
• Uterine distortion or pathology preventing even distribution of copper ions or fundal placement of IUD
• Immunocompromise (chemotherapy, uncontrolled diabetes, AIDS, leukemia, IV drug use, systemic steroid therapy)
• Known or suspected uterine or cervical cancer
• Severe anemia (relative contraindication)

INITIATING METHOD

• Requires insertion by trained professional
• May be inserted at any time in cycle when pregnancy can be ruled out; lowest overall rates of removal are when insertion is at midcycle
➤ • Early expulsion rates lower if avoid insertion during menses
• May be inserted immediately after delivery of the placenta or prior to discharge from hospital after delivery
• Await complete uterine involution postpartum or following second or third trimester loss
• May be inserted immediately after first trimester loss if infection can be ruled out
• One unit may be removed and a second unit inserted at the same visit
• Test for cervical infection, if indicated. Rule out BV (treat prior to insertion)

INSERTION TIPS

• Reconfirm formal consent
• Give NSAIDs one hour prior to insertion (be sure patient is not pregnant)
• Routine antibiotic prophylaxis is not warranted; AHA requires **no** antibiotic treatment for women at risk for bacterial endocarditis
• Recheck position, size and mobility of uterus prior to insertion
• Collect specimens for infection tests, if not done prior to insertion (including vaginal wet mount)
• Cleanse upper vaginal cervix thoroughly with antiseptic

- In some instances provide cervical anesthesia with paracervical block, or lidocaine gel to endocervix and 1/2 cc lidocaine injected into tenaculum site. Paracervical block may ⬅ cause more pain than it prevents
- Place tenaculum to stabilize cervix and straighten uterine axis
- Sound uterus to fundus; may hold sound as pencil when entering internal os to limit uterine perforation risk
- See Figure 25.1 below for copper IUD insertion directions
- Trim strings to about 2" (5 cm) and tuck around cervix. Avoid cutting strings too short or too long. Other clinicians trim strings to 1 - 1.5" (3-4 cm)

Figure 25.1 How to insert a Copper IUD

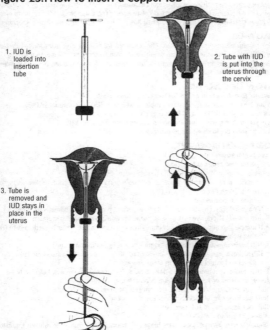

1. IUD is loaded into insertion tube

2. Tube with IUD is put into the uterus through the cervix

3. Tube is removed and IUD stays in place in the uterus

[Speroff L, Darney P. A clinical guide for contraception. 2nd ed. Baltimore: Williams & Wilkins, 1996:215.]

INSTRUCTIONS FOR PATIENT

- Give patient trimmed IUD strings to learn what to check for after menses each month
- Advise patients to return if any symptoms of pregnancy, infection or IUD loss develop:

PAINS: "Early IUD Warning Signs"	
P	Period late (pregnancy); abnormal spotting or bleeding
A	Abdominal pain, pain with intercourse
I	Infection exposure (STI); abnormal vaginal discharge
N	Not feeling well, fever, chills
S	String missing, shorter or longer

- Counsel patient on anticipated menstrual changes. Take NSAIDs prophylactically for first 2-3 days of next 3 menses or even starting just before menses (eg, Ibuprofen 200-400 mg orally every 4-6 hours starting at beginning of menstrual flow). Contact provider if bleeding bothersome

FOLLOW-UP

- Have patient return for post insertion check about 2 1/2 months after insertion to rule out partial expulsion or other problems requiring removal (before end of 3 month warranty). Many clinicians prefer 1 month return visit and then at 2.5 months if any problems. ◄—
- Routine annual well-woman exams

FOLLOW-UP CHECKLIST
Questions to ask women using IUD on each return visit:

- Do you have any questions about/or problems with your IUD? (Remember PAINS)
- Can you feel your IUD strings? Have they changed in length?
- Have you or your partner had any new partners since your last visit?
- When do you plan to start your next pregnancy?

PROBLEM MANAGEMENT
Uterine perforation:

- All perforations start at insertion
- Clinical signs: pain, vaginal bleeding, rapid pulse
- Perforation made by uterine sound usually occurs in midline posterior uterine wall when there is marked flexion
  - Remove uterine sound
  - If no bleeding seen, stable BP and pulse, patient pain free and hematocrit stable for next several hours, she may be sent home. Provide alternate contraception
  - If any persistent pain or signs of other organ damage, take or refer immediately to OR for exploratory surgery
- If IUD perforates acutely, gently attempt removal by pulling on strings
  - If resistance encountered, stop and send to OR for immediate laparoscopic IUD removal and exploration for any other damage
- If IUD perforation noted at later date, arrange for laparoscopic removal electively

Spotting, frequent or heavy bleeding, hemorrhage, anemia

- Rule out pregnancy. If pregnant, rule out ectopic pregnancy
- Rule out infection, especially if post-coital bleeding
- Rule out expulsion of IUD (see below)
- Assess for anemia by lab test
- If anemic or experiences excessive blood loss, check IUD placement to rule out expulsion, provide iron supplement in addition to dealing with cause
- Offer NSAIDs every month to reduce bleeding
- Consider replacement with hormonal IUD

Cramping and/or pain
- Rule out pregnancy, infection, IUD expulsion
- Offer NSAIDs with menses or just before menses every month to reduce cramping
- Consider IUD removal and use of hormonal IUD or another method if problem persists

Expulsion
- Rule out pregnancy
- Probe endocervical canal for IUD - Remove if present. May replace immediately if patient not pregnant

Strings not felt
- Check vagina for strings. Assess string length. If normal, reassure and re-instruct patient how to feel for strings
- If strings missing, perform pregnancy test and select next step below according to outcome

Missing strings in non-pregnant patients
- Twist cytobrush inside cervix to snag strings which may have become snarled in canal
- Examine cervix with uterine sound or visualize canal thru endocervical speculum
- If IUD in endocervix, remove and offer to replace
- If IUD in cervical canal, after paracervical block, attempt to remove with alligator forceps or refer for ultrasound to localize prior to attempted removal (provide interim birth control). Avoid use of IUD hook unless removing Lippes Loop IUD. In non-pregnant patients, removal may also be done under direct hysteroscopic visualization
- Often can locate IUD with ultrasound. If in place may do nothing. If removal necessary, may remove with ultrasound guidance

Missing strings in pregnant patients
- Rule out ectopic pregnancy: 5-8% of all failures with the copper IUD are ectopic
- If intrauterine pregnancy, obtain ultrasound to verify IUD in situ
- If IUD is in uterus, advise patient she is at increased risk for preterm labor but reassure her that fetus is not at increased risk for birth defects. May remove IUD at surgery if patient desires elective abortion. Otherwise, plan for removal at delivery
- Reconfirm formal consent

Pregnancy with visible strings
- Visible strings in first trimester: advise removal of IUD to reduce risk of spontaneous abortion and infection
- Visible strings later in pregnancy: order ultrasound to rule out placenta previa and to localize IUD. IUD removal may not be recommended
- Patient having miscarriage: Remove IUD. Consider antibiotics for 7 days

Infection with IUD use
- *BV or candidiasis:* treat routinely
- *Trichomoniasis:* treat and reassess IUD candidacy. Consider recommending removal
- *Cervicitis or PID:* advise IUD removal. Give first dose of antibiotics to achieve adequate serum levels before removing IUD. If patient refuses removal, provide thorough documentation and consider having process witnessed
- *Actinomycosis:* Culture of assymptomatic women without an IUD AND of women with an IUD both find that 3-4% are positive for Actinomyces *[Lippes, J Am J Obstet Gyn-1999; 180-2 65-9]*. Often suggested by Pap smear report of "Actinomycosis-like organisms". True upper tract infection with this organism is very serious and requires at least prolonged IV antibiotic therapy with penicillin. However, less than half of women with such Pap smear reports have actinomyces and those that do usually have asymptomatic colonization only. Examine patient for any signs of PID (it can be unilateral). If patient has no clinical evidence of upper tract involvement, 3 major options are available: (continued on next page)

1. Conservative. Annual pap smears only. Advise patient to return as needed or if she develops PID symptoms *or*
2. Treat with antibiotic (penicillin G or a tetracycline) and repeat Pap smear *or*
3. Remove IUD and repeat Pap smear in 1 month. Reinsert if colonization cleared

REMOVAL

Indications: Expelling IUD, infection, expired IUD, complications with IUD, anemia, no longer candidate for IUD, patient request.
Procedure: Grasp the strings close to external os and steadily retract until IUD removed.
Complications

- Embedded IUD: Gentle rotation of strings may free IUD. If still stuck, may use alligator forceps removal (see Missing strings). Hysteroscopic removal may be indicated in rare cases. Some clinicians routinely give paracervical block before any uterine instrumentation but usually this is NOT necessary or recommended
- Broken strings: Remove IUD with alligator forceps

FERTILITY AFTER USE

Rapid return to baseline fertility

PROGESTERONE IUD (Progestasert® System)

DESCRIPTION

T-shaped IUD placed into uterine cavity releases 65 micrograms of progesterone a day from vertical limb of IUD. The "T" is made of an ethylene vinyl acetate copolymer, containing 38 mg of progesterone and barium sulfate (for visibility on X-rays); the vertical arm is 36 mm long and the horizontal arms are 32 mm wide. It has blue-black strings, one of which ends 9 cm from top of T, to help provider reconfirm correct placement.

EFFECTIVENESS *(Trussell J, Contraceptive Technology, 1998)*

- Approved for one year of contraceptive protection (18 months in France)
Perfect use failure rate in first year: 1.5% (See Table 13.2, p. 36)
Typical use failure rate in first year: 2.0%

MECHANISM

Causes cervical mucus to become thicker, inhibiting the sperm from reaching upper reproductive tract of woman. Changes in uterotubal fluid impair sperm migration. Endometrial suppression occurs; likelihood of implantation decreased even if ovum has been fertilized. Slight anovulatory effect.

COST in 1995

Setting	Managed Care	Public Sector
Device	$82/year	$82/year
Insertion	207/year	62/year
Removal	70/year	10/year

(Trussell, 1995; Smith, 1993)
Special Cost Savings Programs:

- 3-month warranty: Manufacturer offers to replace any unit that is lost or must be removed within the first 3 months of use.

ADVANTAGES

Menstrual
- May decrease menstrual blood loss (on average)
- Decreases the incidence and intensity of dysmenorrhea

Sexual/psychological
- Convenient: provides spontaneity in sexual activity. Requires no action at time of intercourse
- Reduced fear of pregnancy may make intercourse more pleasurable

Cancers, tumors and masses: May reduce risk of endometrial cancer

Other:
- Rapid return of fertility
- Convenient: single insertion and monthly string check provides 1 year protection
- Private: partner usually not aware of IUD
- May reduce risk of PID

DISADVANTAGES

Menstrual: Progestin effects; spotting and amenorrhea rates increase

Sexual/psychological: Same as copper IUD, p. 79

Cancer, tumors, and masses: None

Other: Same as copper IUD, p. 79

COMPLICATIONS: Same as copper IUD plus persistent ovarian follicular cysts (unusual)

CANDIDATES FOR USE
- Same as copper IUD except some differences in prescribing precautions
- Previous ectopic pregnancy precludes use of Progestasert ⟵

PRESCRIBING PRECAUTIONS: Same as copper IUD except for the following:
- The progesterone IUD *may* be used in women with:
  - Heavier menstrual bleeding and/or dysmenorrhea
  - Uterus sounding to depth of 10 cm
  - Copper allergy or Wilson's disease
- The progesterone IUD may *not* be used in women with diabetes or history of ectopic pregnancy

INITIATING METHOD: See manufacturer's instructions for details about insertion procedures

INSTRUCTIONS FOR PATIENTS
- Same as copper IUD, need to advise patient to expect progestin effects on bleeding

FOLLOW-UP: Same as Copper IUD, p. 82

PROBLEM MANAGEMENT: Same as copper IUD except for the following:
Counseling: Counsel the patient about the effects of progestin on the menstrual cycle
Amenorrhea
- Reassure that amenorrhea due to atrophy of endometrium and uterine vascular changes is to be expected and is not harmful; she is almost certainly not pregnant
- Perform pregnancy test if other signs or symptoms of pregnancy exist or patient concerned
- If concern persists, remove IUD

Severe pain in lower abdomen
- If due to ectopic pregnancy or any other acute gynecologic pathology, treat or refer
- If ovarian cyst(s), IUD may remain in place; reassure that cysts usually regress without surgery. See the patient again in several days for pain and in 3 weeks to 2 months to be sure that cysts are resolving
- If pain is due to other cause, treat or refer

FERTILITY AFTER USE: Immediate and excellent return of fertility

LEVONORGESTREL INTRAUTERINE SYSTEM (Mirena®)

DESCRIPTION

T-shaped intrauterine contraceptive placed within uterine cavity that releases 20 micrograms/day of levonorgestrel from its vertical reservoir. Serum levels of levonorgestrel peak at 25% of the level in POP users taking Ovrette; levels lower than with Norplant. Mirena product information, ordering and reimbursement questions: 1-866-647-3646 (toll free)

EFFECTIVENESS *(Trussell J. Contraceptive Technology, 1998)*

- Active for at least 5 years
- ***Perfect use failure rate in first year:*** < 0.1% (See Table 13.2, p. 36)
- ***Typical use failure rate in first year:*** < 0.1%
- ***5-year failure rate:*** < 0.7%

MECHANISM

Levonorgestrel causes cervical mucus to become thicker, so sperm can not enter upper reproductive tract and do not reach ovum. Changes in uterotubal fluid also impair sperm migration. Alteration of the endometrium prevents implantation of fertilized ovum. This IUD has some anovulatory effect (5-15% of treatment cycles) ◄

COST: $300-400 (Average wholesale price $395)

ADVANTAGES

Menstrual:
- Menorrhagia generally improves (90% vs. 50% with COCs and 30% with PG inhibitors). This may decrease need for hysterectomy for leiomyomata or DUB ◄
- Dysmenorrhea generally improves
- After 3 to 6 months of menstrual irregularities (mostly spotting), Mirena decreases menstrual blood loss more than 70% (97% reduction in menstrual blood loss in one study
- Amenorrhea develops in approximately 20% of users ◄

Sexual/psychological:
- Convenient: permits spontaneous sexual activity. Requires no action at time of intercourse
- Reduced fear of pregnancy can make sex more pleasurable

Cancers, tumors and masses: May have protective effect against endometrial cancer

Other:
- Safe, extremely effective; More effective than female sterilization
- Anemia improves
- May decrease a woman's risk for PID (RR: 0.6 compared to women using no method)
- Used as the progestin by women on HRT in countries where Mirena IUS is available
- Used as treatment for menorrhagia
- Decreased risk for ectopic pregnancy
- May reduce menstrual symptoms in women with uterine fibroids or adenomyosis, possible reducing need for hysterectomy ◄
- May reduce occurrence of benign endometrial polyps in breast cancer patients taking tamoxifen (new UK data) ◄

DISADVANTAGES

Menstrual: (Removal for any bleeding problem in first year: 7.6%)
- Number of bleeding days is higher than normal for first few months and lower than normal after 3 to 6 months of using levonorgestrel intrauterine system
- Amenorrhea (a negative if not explained, a positive for a woman if explained well in advance) occurs in about 20% of women at one year of use ◄

Sexual/psychological: Same as other intrauterine contraceptives except when spotting and bleeding may interfere with sexual activity

Other:
- Offers no protection against STIs, except perhaps PID
- May be expelled (median expulsion rate of 19 studies in product monograph 4.8%) ◄
- Persistent unruptured follicles may cause ovarian enlargement/cysts. Most cysts regress spontaneously
- Headaches, acne, mastalgia during first months ◄
- Pain during or for one day or so after insertion or removal

COMPLICATIONS: See 2001 WHO Medical Eligibility Criteria - Appendix: A1 - A8
- PID risk transiently increased after insertion; Large painful ovarian cysts
- Allergy to levonorgestrel and perforation (rare)

CANDIDATES FOR USE
- Women wanting long-term contraception but wanting to avoid tubal sterilization
- Same as copper IUD except that levonorgestrel intrauterine contraceptive can be used in women with heavy menses, cramps or anemia
- Menopausal women using ERT, with intact uteri, who are unable to tolerate other oral progestins. These women may be able to get protection from endometrial carcinoma by using a levonorgestrel intrauterine contraceptive *[Raudaskoski, 1995]*

PRESCRIBING PRECAUTIONS: See WHO Precautions in Appendix: A-1 - A-8)

INITIATING METHOD See Figure 25.2, pages 88-91
- *The one-hand insertion technique is different from current IUDs. Training (call 1-866-LNG-IUS1) is highly recommended before inserting Mirena* ◄
- Usually inserted within 7 days of onset of menses
- If no pregnancy exists, it may be possible to insert an intrauterine contraceptive at other times of cycle
- Insertion tube is wider than for other intrauterine contraceptives; may occasionally need to dilate cervix
- A local anesthetic (paracervical block) may be required in some patients
- Counsel in advance to expect menstrual cycle changes
- Advise NSAIDs for post-insertion discomfort. If pain persists, she must return

INSTRUCTIONS FOR PATIENT: Similar to copper intrauterine contraceptive, p. 82

FOLLOW-UP
- Have your periods ceased or become sporadic?
- Have you experienced any bleeding or spotting or had heavy or prolonged bleeding?
- Have you noticed any change in the string length?
- Have you had any lower abdominal pain?
- Have you experienced headaches, blurred vision, or dizziness?

PROBLEM MANAGEMENT: Similar to Progestasert, see p. 85

FERTILITY AFTER USE
- Immediate and excellent return of fertility

Figure 25.2 How to insert Mirena IUS ◄

Preparation for insertion:

- Confirm that the patient understands the method and alternatives and has signed a consent form

- Examine the patient to establish the size and position of the uterus to detect cervicitis or other genital contraindications and to exclude pregnancy

- Obtain cervical cultures, perform a pregnancy test and give antibiotic prophylaxis if indicated

- Use aseptic technique during insertion

- Administer oral analgesics if needed

- Cleanse the cervix and vagina with an antiseptic solution

- Administer paracervical block if needed

- Grasp the upper lip of the cervix with a tenaculum and apply gentle traction to align the cervical canal with the uterine cavity

- Carefully sound the uterus to measure its depth and to check the patency of the cervix. If you encounter cervical stenosis, use dilatation, not force, to overcome resistance

- The uterus should sound to a depth of 6 to 9 cm. Insertion of MIRENA into a uterine cavity less than 6.0 cm by sounding may increase the incidence of expulsion, bleeding, pain, perforation, and possibly, pregnancy.

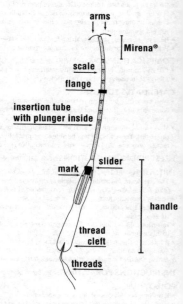

MIRENA® and Inserter

Insertion Procedure:

1)
- Open the sterile package

- Place sterile gloves on your hands

- Pick up the inserter containing MIRENA®

- Carefully release the threads from behind the slider, so that they hang freely

- Make sure that the slider is in the furthest position away from you (positioned at the top of the handle nearest the IUS)

- While looking at the insertion tube, check that the arms of the system are horizontal. If not, align them on a sterile surface or with sterile gloved fingers

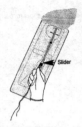

Checking that the arms of the system are horizontal

---

2)
- Pull on both threads to draw the MIRENA® system into the insertion tube (figure a)

- Note that the knobs at the end of the arms now cover the open end of the inserter (figure b)

a) MIRENA® system being drawn into the insertion tube

b) The knobs at the ends of the arms

---

3)
- Fix the threads tightly in the cleft at end of the handle

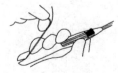

Threads are fixed tightly in the cleft

4)
• Set the flange to the depth measured by the sound

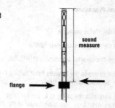

sound
measure

flange

The sound measure

5)
• MIRENA® is now ready to be inserted. Hold the slider firmly in the furthermost position (at the top of the handle). Grasp the cervix with the tenaculum and apply gentle traction to align the cervical canal with the uterine cavity. Gently insert the inserter into the cervical canal and advance the insertion tube into the uterus until the flange is situated at a distance of about 1.5-2 cm from the external cervical os to give sufficient space for the arms to open. **NOTE: Do not force the inserter**

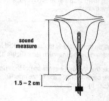

sound
measure

1.5 – 2 cm

Flange adjusted to sound depth

6)
• While holding the inserter steady release the arms of MIRENA® by pulling the slider back until the top of the slider reaches the mark (raised horizontal line on the handle)

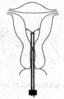

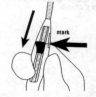

mark

The arms of the MIRENA® being released

Pulling the slider back to reach the mark

7)
- Push the inserter gently into the uterine cavity until the flange touches the cervix. MIRENA® should now be in the fundal position

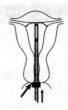

MIRENA® in the fundal position

---

8)
- Holding the inserter firmly in position release MIRENA® by pulling the slider down all the way. The threads will be released automatically

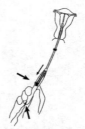

Releasing MIRENA® and withdrawing the inserter

---

9)
- Remove the inserter from the uterus. Cut the threads to leave about 2-3 cm visible outside the cervix

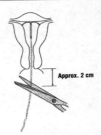

Approx. 2 cm

Cutting the threads

DESCRIPTION

Progestin-only pills (POPs) are also known as mini-pills. POPs contain only a progestin and are taken daily with no hormone-free days. POPs have lower progestin doses than combined pills. Each tablet of Micronor and Nor-QD contains 0.35 mg norethindrone. Each tablet of Ovrette has 0.075 mg of norgestrel.

EFFECTIVENESS *(Trussell J., Contraceptive Technology 1998)*
Perfect use failure rate in first year: 0.5% (See Table 13.2, p. 36)
(if 200 women take POPs for 1 year, only 1 will become pregnant in the first year of perfect use)
Typical use failure rate in first year: 5.0%

MECHANISM

Thickens cervical mucus to prevent sperm entry into upper reproductive tract (major mechanism). Effect short lived - requires punctual dosing. Other mechanisms include ovulation suppression (in about 50% of cycles), thin, atrophic endometrium which inhibits implantation; and slowed tubal mobility

COST *[Trussel, 1995; Smith, 1993]*

Setting	Managed-Care (1995)	Public Provider (1995)
Pills	$21.00/cycle	$17.70/cycle
Office Visit	$38.00	$16.56

ADVANTAGES
Menstrual:
  • Decreased menstrual blood loss. Amenorrhea (10% of women overall)
  • Decreased menstrual cramps and pain
  • Decrease in ovulatory pain (Mittelschmerz) in cycles when ovulation suppressed
Sexual/physiological:
  • May enhance sexual enjoyment due to diminished fear of pregnancy
  • No disruption at time of intercourse; facilitates spontaneity
Cancers, tumors and masses:
  • Possible protection against endometrial cancer
Other:
  • Rapid return to fertility
  • Possible reduction in PID risk due to cervical mucus thickening
  • Good option for women who cannot use estrogen but want to take pills

DISADVANTAGES
Menstrual:
  • Irregular menses ranging from amenorrhea to increased days of spotting and bleeding but with reduced overall blood loss

Sexual/psychological:
- Spotting and bleeding may interfere with sexual activity
- Intermittent amenorrhea may raise concerns about pregnancy
- Possible increase in depression, anxiety, irritability, fatigue or other mood changes but often POPs reduce risk of these disorders

Cancers, tumors and masses:
- May be associated with slightly higher risk of persistent ovarian follicles

Other:
- Must take pill at same time each day (more than 3-hour delay considered by some clinicians to be equivalent to a "missed pill")
- Effect on cervical mucus decreases after 22 hours and is gone after 27 hours
- No protection against STIs. Must use condom if at risk

COMPLICATIONS
- Allergy to progestin pill is rare
- Amenorrheic, Latina, breast-feeding women who had gestational diabetes may be at higher risk of developing overt diabetes in first year of use *[Kjos, 1998]*

CANDIDATES FOR USE
- Virtually every woman who can take pills on a daily basis can be a candidate for POPs, although the relatively high failure rates of these pills compared to other hormonal methods makes them less attractive. See PRESCRIBING PRECAUTIONS below
- POPs are particularly good for women with contraindications to or side effects from estrogen or higher-dose progestins:
- Women with personal history of thrombosis or strong family history of VTE
- Recently postpartum women
- Women who are exclusively breast-feeding (until lactation is well established)
- Smokers over age 35
- Women who had or fear chloasma, worsening migraine headaches, hypertriglyceridemia or other estrogen-related side effects
- Women with hypertension, coronary artery disease or cerebrovascular disease (see WHO Precautions in Appendix)

PRESCRIBING PRECAUTIONS
Progestin-only pills can be used by all women willing and able to take daily pills except:
- Suspected or demonstrated pregnancy (although there are no proven harmful effects for the fetus)
- Personal history of breast cancer
- Hepatic failure, jaundice
- Inability to absorb sex steroids from gastrointestinal tract (active colitis, etc.)
- Taking medications that increase hepatic clearance (rifampin, certain anticonvulsants, St. Johns Wort or griseofulvin). Efficacy in face of Orlistat and other fat-binding agents is not well studied

MEDICAL ELIGIBILITY CHECKLIST: Ask the client the questions below. If she answers NO to ALL of the questions, then she CAN use POPs if she wants. If she answers YES to a question below, follow the instructions; in some cases she can still use POPs

1. Do you think you are pregnant?

☐ No ☐ Yes Assess if pregnant. If she might be pregnant, give her condoms or spermicide to use until reasonably sure that she is not pregnant. Then she can start POPs

2. Do you have or have you ever had breast cancer? (See page A4)

☐ No ☐ Yes Do not provide POPs. Help her choose a method without hormones

3. Do you have jaundice, severe cirrhosis of the liver, acute liver infection or tumor? (Are her eyes or skin unusually yellow?) (See page A5)

☐ No ☐ Yes Perform physical exam and arrange lab tests or refer. If she has serious active liver disease (jaundice, painful or enlarged liver, viral hepatitis, liver tumor), do not provide POPs. Refer for care. Help her choose a method without hormones

4. Do you have vaginal bleeding that is unusual for you? (See page A3)

☐ No ☐ Yes If she is not pregnant but has unexplained vaginal bleeding that suggests an underlying medical condition, can provide POPs since neither the underlying condition nor its assessment will be affected. Assess and treat any underlying condition as appropriate, or refer. Reassess POP use based on findings

5. Are you taking medicine for seizures? Taking rifampin (rifampicin), griseofulvin or aminoglutethimide? St. Johns Wort? ◄──

☐ No ☐ Yes If she is taking phenytoin, carbamazepine, barbiturate, or primidone for seizures or rifampin, griseofulvin, aminoglutethamide or St. John's Wort provide condoms or spermicide to use each exposure along with POPs. If she prefers or if she is on long-term treatment, help her choose another method that is more effective, such as DMPA

6. Do you have problems with severe diarrhea from Crohn's disease or other bowel disorders? Or are you using medications that block fat absorption?

☐ No ☐ Yes Help her choose a non-oral method of birth control

7. If patient < 1 year since delivering and had gestational diabetes, ask is she breast-feeding?

☐ No ☐ Yes Counsel that she may be at higher risk for developing glucose intolerance or overt diabetes. Consider IUD or COCs, if feasible

SPECIAL SITUATIONS

History of pregnancy while using POPs correctly:
- Consider longer acting, higher dose progestin methods (DMPA, Norplant)
- Switch to estrogen containing methods or IUDs
- Continue POPs but add condoms or other backup with every act of coitus

Use with a broad-spectrum antibiotic such as tetracycline or erythromycin:
- Few studies support antibiotic's role in contraceptive failure, but most studies focus on COCs. Some clinicians encourage backup for first 1-2 weeks, others for full duration of antibiotic use. Explain conflicting advice now being given to women, your own opinion, and let patient decide whether to use backup method. **More discussion, go to:** www.managingcontraception.com/questions_new/oral/g-a_or_06-12.html ◄── 95

INITIATING METHOD

- *New starts:* Offer condoms either for back-up or for use should patient stop POP
- *Post-partum:* May initiate immediately regardless of breast-feeding status
  Note: WHO and IPPF are concerned about hypothetical impact of progestin on breast milk production in third world countries with poor maternal nutrition and recommend delaying initiation until six weeks postpartum. In this case, strongly encourage abstinence or condom use until 6 weeks postpartum
- *After miscarriage or abortion:* Start immediately
- *Menstruating women:* Start on menses if possible. May initiate anytime in cycle if woman is not pregnant, but recommend at least 1-week back-up barrier method.
- *Switching from IUD, COCs, DMPA, to POPs:* start immediately. Need for back-up ◄—— depends on previous method used: **IUD:** start immediately, backup for 2 weeks; Creinin - 48 hours minimum; others say no backup. **COCs:** start immediately if cycle of hormonally active pills completed; backup not necessary if no pill-free interval
  DMPA: start immediately if switching at or before next DMPA injection due in which case no backup is necessary.

INSTRUCTIONS FOR PATIENT

- Take one pill daily at *same* time each day until end of pack. Start next pack the next day
- If at risk for infection, use condoms with every act of intercourse
- If you miss a pill by more than 3 hours from regular time, take the missed pill(s) and use backup contraception for 7 days. Consider using emergency contraception if intercourse in past 3-5 days

FOLLOW-UP

- How many pills do you typically miss or are late taking per week? Per pack?
- Have you missed any pills in last 3 days? (candidate for EC)
- Have you missed any periods or experienced any symptoms of pregnancy?
- What has you menstrual bleeding been like?
- Have you had any increase in your headaches or change in vision?
- When do you plan to start your next pregnancy?

PROBLEM MANAGEMENT

- *Amenorrhea:* Rule out pregnancy with first episode or whenever symptoms of pregnancy noted. Otherwise, amenorrhea is not harmful when women take progestin-only pills.
- *Irregular bleeding:* Rule out STIs, pregnancy, cancer. If not at risk and no evidence of underlying pathology, reassure patient. Offer 3-day course of high dose NSAIDS
- *Heavy bleeding:* Rule out STIs, pregnancy, cancer. If no evidence of underlying pathology, rule out clinically significant anemia. Trial of 3 days high dose NSAIDS. If fails, may need estrogen-containing contraceptives (addition of physiologic doses ERT only may compromise cervical mucus barrier) or other non-hormonal methods of contraception.
- *Abdominal pain:* Consider pelvic pathology (ectopic pregnancy, torsion, PID) and refer for treatment. If ovarian cyst is cause, it may be managed conservatively. Progestin slows follicular atresia. Recheck in 6 weeks and anytime her symptoms worsen.
- *Severe headaches:* If new onset or worsening of headaches, blurred vision with flashing lights, loss of vision, trouble moving or speaking - stop POPs and seek immediate help

FERTILITY AFTER USE

Fertility returns to its baseline levels promptly after discontinuation of progestin only pills

DESCRIPTION

Each active pill in the 28-day cycle contains an estrogen and
a progestin. Ethinyl estradiol (EE) is the most commonly
used estrogen; it is in most 50 µg pills and all of the sub-50
µg formulations. Mestranol, which must be metabolized to
EE to become biologically active, is found in two 50 µg formulations (rarely prescribed).
In the conversion of mestranol to EE, 30% of the hormone is lost, so 50 µg mestranol is
equivalent to 35 µg EE in efficacy. At least 3 progestins are used in the different pill
formulations. All packs have 21 active combined pills, with or without 7 additional pills
(usually placebo pills). Monophasic formulations contain active pills with the same amount
of hormones in each tablet. Multiphasic formulations contain active pills with varying
amounts of progestin and/or estrogen in the active pills of the cycle. One formulation
(Mircette) has the traditional 21 days of active pills followed by 2 days of placebo pills and
5 days of pills with 10 µg EE alone. As this book went to press, Cyclessa, a triphasic OC
with increasing levels of desogestrel (see p. A-18) and Yasmin, a monophasic pill with
antimineralocorticoid activity were approved by the FDA.

EFFECTIVENESS *[Trussell J, Contraceptive Technology, 1998]*

Perfect use failure rate in first year: 0.1% (of every 1,000 women who take pills for 1 year,
1 will become pregnant in the first year use) (See Table 13.2, p. 36)
Typical use failure rate in first year: 5%

MECHANISM

Suppresses ovulation (90% to 95% of time). Also causes thickening of cervical mucus, which
blocks sperm penetration and entry into the upper reproductive track. Thin, asynchronous
endometrium inhibits implantation. Tubal and endometrial motility slowed.

COST *[Trussell, 1995; Smith, 1993]*

	Managed-Care Setting	Public Provider Setting
COCs	$21/cycle	$17.70/cycle (much lower in some clinics)
Office Visit	$38	$16.56 (lower in many clinics)

- Cost of one cycle: from a few dollars to more than $50. Most cost $20-$42/cycle in pharmacies.
- Costs differ from region to region, and pills with more estrogen often cost more.
- Generic brands are generally less expensive. They are not required to have clinical testing;
  they must only prove blood level equivalency (80–125% of parent compound's blood levels)

ADVANTAGES

Menstrual:
- Decreased blood loss, decreased menstrual cramps/pain and more predictable menses
- Eliminates ovulation pain (Mittelschmerz)
- Can use to manipulate timing and frequency of menses (see Choice of COC, p. 104 and 108)
- Reduces risk of internal hemorrhage from ovulation (especially important in women
  with bleeding diatheses or anticoagulation)

Sexual/psychological:
- No disruption at time of intercourse; more spontaneous activity
- Enhanced sexual enjoyment due to diminished risk of pregnancy
- Potential psychological benefits from women being able to control, skip or time menses

Cancers/tumors/masses:

- Decreased risk for epithelial **ovarian cancer** (clearly demonstrated for 50 µg and higher dose pills); COC users for 5 years have 50% reduction in risk; users for 10 years have 80% reduction
- Protection extends for 30 years beyond last pill use; Significant reduction in risk also seen in high risk women
- Decreased risk for **endometrial cancer** (clearly demonstrated for 30 µg and higher dose pills)
  - COC users for 1 year have 20% reduction in risk; users for 4 years have 60% reduction
  - Protection lasts for 30 years after last pill *[Ness, AmJEpidemiol-2000]* ←
  - Particularly important for PCOS women, obese women, and perimenopausal women
- *Breast masses:* 25% reduction in all *benign breast disease* (including fibroadenomas)
- Decreased risk of death from **colorectal cancer** seen in current COC users and in women who used COCs within the last 10 years *[Berel 1999]*
- Decreased risk of corpus luteum cysts and hemorrhagic corpus luteum cysts

Other:

- Reduces risk of PID and ectopic pregnancy
- Treatment for acne, hirsutism and other androgen excess states
- Reduced vasomotor symptoms in perimenopausal women
- Increased bone mineral density when pills with 35 micrograms of estrogen used by women ← in their 40s have been found to reduce postmenopausal hip fractures *[Michaelsson-1998; Lancet, 353:1481-1484]*. 20 mcg pills probably have similar benefit

DISADVANTAGES

Menstrual:

- Spotting, particularly during first few cycles and with inconsistent use
- Scant or missed menses possible, but not clinically significant
- Post-pill amenorrhea (lasts up to 6 months). Uncommon and usually in women with history of irregular periods prior to taking pills

Sexual/psychological:

- Decreased libido is possible, but unusual
- Mood changes, depression, anxiety, irritability, fatigue may develop while on COCs
- Rule out other causes before implicating COCs
- Daily pill taking may be stressful (especially if privacy is an issue)

Cancers/tumors/masses:

- *Breast cancer:*
  - Large meta-analysis found no statistically significant overall increase in COC users,
→ even among women with strong family history. However, recent Mayo Clinic study of women with affected first degree relatives, found that OCs may further amplify risk *[Grabrick, JAMA - 2000]*
→ COCs do not cause breast cancer; but these may be a detection bias causing slightly more breast cancers to be diagnosed in women on pills (2-3 cancers per 100,000 women under 35)
→ Breast cancer, if diagnosed in women on COCs or after COC use, is less likely to be metastatic *[Ness, Am J Epidemiol-2000]*
  - *Cervical cancer:*
    - No consistent increased risk seen for squamous cell cervical carcinoma (85% of all cervical cancer) after controlling for confounding variables, such as number of sex partners. Risk of a relatively uncommon type of cervical cancer, adenocarcinoma, is increased 60%, but no extra screening required
- *Hepatocellular adenoma:* risk increased among COC users (especially ≥ 50 µg formulations).

Risk of hepatic carcinoma not increased, even in populations with high prevalence of Hepatitis B

Other:

- No protection against STIs, including HIV. Must use safer sex practices, including condoms
- Nausea and vomiting, especially in first few cycles
- Breast tenderness, especially in first few cycles
- Headaches: may increase in frequency and/or intensity
- Increased varicosities, chloasma, capillary spiders
- Daily dosing may be difficult for some women
- Weight gain reported by some COC users, but average weight gain no different among COC users than placebo users (see NOTE below)
- Bone mineralization in late teens may not be maximal in COC users (COC users increased 1.5% versus 2.9% in controls) *[Cromer, 1996]*
- See COMPLICATIONS section below
- NOTE: Medical problems and symptom complaints are frequently attributed by patients and providers to COC use. While some women may be particularly sensitive to sex steroids, a recent placebo-controlled study found that the incidence of all of the frequently mentioned hormone-related side effects was not significantly different in the COC group than it was in the placebo group *[Redmond, 1999]*

"SIDE EFFECT"	Triphasic Norgestimate/EE (N=228) N (%)	Placebo (N=234) N (%)	p-value
Headache	42 (18.4)	48 (20.5)	0.639
Nausea	29 (12.7)	21 (9.0)	0.231
Dysmenorrhea	23 (10.1)	21 (9.0)	.752
Breast pain	21 (9.2)	11 (4.7)	.067
Abdominal pain	13 (5.7)	9 (3.9)	.270
Back pain	13 (5.7)	8 (3.4)	.597
Vomiting	8 (3.5)	6 (2.6)	.597
Breast enlargement	6 (2.6)	3 (1.3)	.333
Emotional liability	6 (2.6)	1 (0.4)	.065
Weight gain	5 (2.2)	5 (2.1)	1.000

COMPLICATIONS

- *Venous thromboembolism (VTE)*
  - The risk of VTE with COC use is less than with pregnancy:

No COC use	4-8/100,000 women per year
COC use	10-30/100,000 women per year
Pregnancy	60/100,000 women per year

- DVT risk is associated with dose of estrogen; the risk of VTE in 50 µg pills is greater than 20-35 µg pills. The type of progestin may slightly influence DVT risk; 1996 studies ← demonstrated a two-fold increased risk of DVT in desogestrel and gestodene users. The current COC labeling states that there is an increased DVT risk for women using desogestrel pills. The debate continues-stay tuned. Underlying blood dyscrasias such as Factor V$_{Leiden}$ mutation and Protein S or C abnormalities increase risk of VTE significantly
- *Myocardial infarction (MI) and stroke*
  - There is no increased risk of MI or stroke for young women who are using low-dose COCs who do not smoke, do not have hypertension and do not have migraine headaches with neurological findings
  - Women at risk:
    - Smokers over 35 shouldn't use COCs; all smokers should be encouraged to stop smoking. Smokers over 35 have MI rate of 396 per million COC users per year vs. 88 per million non-COC users per year
    - Hypertension, diabetes, hyperlipidemia or obesity
    - Migraine headaches, new onset headaches (only stroke risk increases)

- Desogestrel and norgestimate have labeling that indicates that decreased androgenicity may decrease risk of MI compared to other progestin formulations (although the supporting data are not conclusive)
- *Hypertension:* 1% of users develop hypertension which (usually) is reversible within 1-3 months of discontinuing COCs. Most users have a very small increase in blood pressure

---

ELEVATED BLOOD PRESSURE: A TEACHABLE MOMENT ◄

Your very quick advice each time you find an elevated blood pressure might include several messages.

1. **Stop smoking.** If you smoke, it is by far the most important step you can take
2. **Exercise regularly. Moderate exercise for 20-30 minutes each day**
3. **Lose weight** (if overweight)
4. **Use salt in moderation**
5. **If you are on antihypertensive medications, take them regularly!**
6. **Work on reducing the stress in your life** (may be difficult and may take time)

- *Neoplasia:* COC users are at higher risk of developing adenocarcinoma of the cervix and hepatic adenomas. Breast cancer risk is neutral except that young women on COCs may develop clinically detectable breast cancer earlier
- *Cholelithiasis/cholecystitis:* higher dose formulations were associated with doubling the risk of symptomatic gallbladder disease
  - Sub-50 mcg formulations may be neutral or have a slightly increased risk
  - Use COCs with caution in women with known gallstones
  - See page 103 #11
- *Visual changes:* Rare cases of retinal thrombosis. Contact lens users may have dry eye— may recommend eye drops or need to switch methods

CANDIDATES FOR USE

- Most healthy reproductive aged women are candidates for COCs.
- For healthy women, the use of COCs is often decided on the basis of a balance of perceived benefits and side effects. Careful counseling can help patient recognize all the health benefits COCs offer and help motivate her to daily COC use.
- Women with conditions listed under prescribing precautions may occasionally be candidates for COC use if the benefits outweigh the risk as discussed in the MEDICAL ELIGIBILITY CHECKLIST section (see p. 101 & Appendix A-1–A-8). However, non-hormonal methods or hormonal methods that do not contain estrogen are generally more appropriate. In addition to medical precautions, real world considerations such as the need for privacy, affordable access to COCs, and the requirement for daily administration need to be considered when evaluating a woman for COC use.

Adolescents

- May be excellent candidates for contraceptive benefits if patient is able to take a pill each day.
- Many of the non-contraceptive effects of OCs are particularly important for adolescent women – e.g. decreased dysmenorrhea (the most common cause of lost days of school and work among women under 25), and decreased acne, hirsutism, or hypoestrogenism due to eating disorders, excessive exercise, stress, etc.
- Failure rates are higher in teens using COCs. Help teens integrate pill taking into daily rituals (tooth brushing, beeper, watch alarm, application of makeup, putting on earrings). Ask teenager how she will create a way to be successful.
- Encourage teens to use condoms if at risk for STIs.

SPECIAL CONSIDERATIONS FOR USE

- Women with medical conditions that improve with COCs may find COCs a particularly attractive contraceptive option. This includes women with endometriosis, menstrual migraine (except those who have migraine with aura or other neurologic symptoms), or iron deficiency anemia, acne, hirsutism, polycystic ovarian syndrome (PCOS), ovarian or endometrial cancer risk factors or eating disorders or activity patterns that increase risk of osteoporosis
- Women whose reproductive health would be improved by ovulation suppression or decreased menstrual blood loss should also use COCs. This includes women who suffer menorrhagia or dysmenorrhea, some anticoagulated women (COCs decrease risk of internal hemorrhage with ovulation and menorrhagia) and women using seizure medication (decrease menorrhagia). Certain anti-seizure medications may lower COC effectiveness
- Women whose quality of life would be improved by reducing frequency of or eliminating menses with continuous COC use: e.g. athletes, women on assignment (military, etc), dancers, women with any demanding schedule or any woman who prefers not menstruating, or women with cyclic depression, headaches or PMS

PRESCRIBING PRECAUTIONS (See 2001 WHO precautions in the Appendix, p. A1-A8 for detailed Medical Eligibility Criteria)

- Thrombophlebitis, thromboembolic disease or history of deep venous thrombosis or pulmonary embolism (unless anticoagulated)
- Family history of multiple family members with multiple unexplained VTE at an early age (eg Factor V_{Leiden})
- Cerebral vascular disease or coronary artery disease
- Current breast cancer (WHO: 4)
- Past breast cancer and no evidence of current disease for 5 years - WHO: 3
- Endometrial carcinoma or other estrogen dependent neoplasia (excluding endometriosis and leiomyoma)
- Unexplained vaginal bleeding suspicious for serious condition (before evaluation) - WHO: 2
- Cholestatic jaundice of pregnancy or jaundice with prior pill use
- Hepatic adenoma or carcinoma or significant hepatic dysfunction
- Smoking after age 35
- Complicated or prolonged diabetes, uncontrolled hypertension, systemic lupus erythematosus
- Severe migraine with neurologic symptoms

MEDICAL ELIGIBILITY CHECKLIST

Ask client the questions below. If she answers NO to ALL of the questions and has no other contraindications, then she can use low-dose COCs if she wants. If she answers YES to a question below, follow the instructions

1. Do you think you are pregnant?

☐ No ☐ Yes Assess if pregnant. If she might be pregnant, give her condoms or spermicide to use until reasonably certain that she is not pregnant. Then she can start COCs. If unprotected sex within past 3 days, consider emergency contraception if she is not pregnant.

2. Do you smoke cigarettes and are you age 35 or older?

☐ No ☐ Yes Urge her to stop smoking. If she is 35 or older and she will not stop smoking, do not provide COCs. Help her choose a method without estrogen.

3. Do you have high blood pressure? (see Appendix, p. A2)

☐ No ☐ Yes *If BP below 140/90, OK to give COCs. If BP is elevated, see Appendix, p. A-3. Consider POPs.*

4. Are you breast-feeding your baby?

☐ No ☐ Yes *No controversy:* Provide the COCs she will use when she stops nursing. Also provide interval contraceptive she may use while nursing her baby. *Some controversy:* Provide COCs and counsel to start when she adds nutrition from other sources (bottle milk or solid foods). Provide interval method. *Controversial,* but supported by clinical studies: may start COCs after lactation well established. Strongly consider POPs while nursing baby ◄──

5. Do you have serious medical problems such as a heart attack, severe chest pain, blood clots, high blood pressure or diabetes? Have you ever had such problems?

☐ No ☐ Yes Do not provide COCs if she reports heart attack or heart disease due to blocked arteries, stroke, blood clots (except superficial clots), severe chest pain with unusual shortness of breath, diabetes for more than 20 years, or damage to vision, kidneys, or nervous system caused by diabetes. Help her choose a method without estrogen. Consider POPs

6. Do you have or have you ever had breast cancer? (see p. A4)

☐ No ☐ Yes Do not provide COCs. Help her choose a method without hormones.

7. Do you often get bad headaches with blurred vision, nausea or dizziness?

☐ No ☐ Yes If she gets migraine headaches and has blurred vision, temporary loss of vision, sees flashing lights or zigzag lines, or has trouble speaking or moving or other neurologic symptoms, do not provide COCs unless she has only menstrual migraines (see choice of COC use, p. 110). Help her choose a method without estrogen. Consider POPs

8. Are you taking medicine for seizures? Are you taking rifampin or griseofulvin?

☐ No ☐ Yes If she has no breakthrough bleeding, she can continue using only the pill. If she is using rifampin or griseofulvin, guide her to DMPA or a non-hormonal method (see p. 105) or strongly encourage condom use. If she is taking phenytoin, carbamazepine, barbiturates, or primidone for seizures, provide condoms to use along with COCs. May also consider raising dose of COCs to 50 µg EE pills, or help her choose another effective method if she is on long-term treatment. She may be able to use 35-µg pills, using breakthrough bleeding as a marker of ovulation control. Some have suggested using condoms for the first 3 months as a backup.

9. Do you have vaginal bleeding that is unusual for you? (see Appendix, p. A3)

☐ No ☐ Yes If she is not likely to be pregnant but has unexplained vaginal bleeding that suggests an underlying medical condition, evaluate condition before initiating pills. Treat as appropriate or refer. Reassess COC use based on findings.

10. Do you have jaundice, cirrhosis of the liver, an acute liver infection or tumor? (Are her eyes or skin unusually yellow?) (see p. A5)

☐ No ☐ Yes If she has serious active liver disease (jaundice, painful or enlarged liver, active viral hepatitis, liver tumor), do not provide COCs. Refer for care as appropriate. Help her choose a method without hormones.

11. Do you have gallbladder disease? Ever had jaundice while taking COCs or during pregnancy?

☐ No ☐ Yes If she has acute gallbladder disease now or takes medicine for gallbladder disease, or if she has had jaundice while using COCs or during pregnancy, do not provide COCs. Consider a method without estrogen. Women with known asymptomatic cholelithiasis or sludge may use COCs with caution.

12. Are you planning surgery that will keep you from walking for a week or more? Have you had a baby in the past 21 days?

☐ No ☐ Yes Help her choose a method without estrogen. If planning surgery or just had a baby, provide COCs for delayed initiation and another interim method.

13. Have you ever gotten pregnant on the pill?

☐ No ☐ Yes Ask about pill-taking habits. Consider longer dosing hormonal methods or shortening or eliminating the pill-free interval while using COCs.

INITIATING METHOD (see INSTRUCTIONS FOR PATIENT, p. 105)

- *Counseling is critical in helping women successfully use the pill*
  - Patients who are counseled well about how to use pills and what side effects may develop are usually better prepared and may be more likely to continue use
- *Timing of initiation* (see Table 27.1, p. 107)
  - **First day of next menstrual period start is generally preferred because no routine backup method is needed**
  - If using Sunday start, recommend back-up method x 7 days.
  - Same day start is quite feasible to help women (especially teens) adapt to COCs
    - If patient not switching from another hormonal method, provide 7 day backup
  - For special cases, see Table 27.1, p. 105
- *Choice of pill*
  - The pill that will work best for the woman is the one that she will take
  - For special situations, some formulations offer advantages over others (see CHOOSING COCs FOR WOMEN IN SPECIAL SITUATIONS, p. 104)
    - In general, use the lowest dose of hormones that will provide pregnancy protection, deliver the non-contraceptive benefits that are important to the woman, and minimize her side effects.
    - Monophasic formulations are preferable if women are interested in controlling cycle lengths or timing by eliminating any or all pill-free intervals for medical indications or personal preference (see Choosing COCs, p. 104)

- Triphasic formulations may be preferable to use to reduce some side effects (such as premenstrual breakthrough bleeding) when it is not desirable to increase hormone levels throughout the entire cycle or when it is desirable to reduce total cycle progestin levels (e.g. acne treatment). There is no definite research indicating ← the superiority of triphasic pills for women with BTB.

- *Choice of pattern of COC use*
  - 28-day cycling: Most common use pattern. Women have monthly withdrawal bleeding during placebo pills
  - *"First day start" each cycle:* Women can start each new pack of pills on first day of menses each cycle, but never use more than 3-5 days of placebos before starting new pack. Beware: This may be confusing
  - *"Bicycling" or "tricycling":* Women skip placebo pills for either 1 or 2 packs and then use the placebo pills and have withdrawal bleeding every 7 weeks (end of 2nd pack) or 10 weeks (end of 3rd pack). **Use monophasic pills** ←
  - You may prescribe 4 packs of low dose monophasic pills omitting the placebo pills. The new pills, *Seasonal*, will be packaged to provide pills in this manner: 84 active pills followed by 6 days of inactive pills.
  - *"Continuous use":* Women take only active pills and have no withdrawal bleeding. Often women must transition through bicycling or tricycling to achieve amenorrhea. Must use monophasic pills
  - *NOTE: the last three options are particularly good for:*
    - Women with menstrually-related problems (menorrhagia, anemia due to any cause, dysmenorrhea, menstrual irregularity, endometriosis, menstrual migraine)
    - Women on medications that reduce COC effectiveness (e.g. anticonvulsants, St. John's Wort)
    - Women who have conceived while on COCs or who forget to take them regularly
    - Women who want to control their cycles for their own convenience
    - Women under 35 who smoke. Smokers have 20% reduction in estrogen (older smokers are not COC candidates)

CHOOSING COCs FOR WOMEN IN SPECIAL SITUATIONS
- *Diabetes and glucose intolerance:* low-dose pills with lower progestin content and low androgenicity to reduce insulin resistance and cardiovascular risks
- *Endometriosis:* relatively strong progestin content helpful to create pseudo-pregnancy state. Continuous use COCs most effective in reducing symptoms
- *Functional ovarian cysts:* higher dose COCs more effective. If using 50 µg formulations, select one with EE for maximum effectiveness
- *Androgen excess states:* all COCs are helpful but pills with higher estrogen/progestin ratios and low androgenicity are preferable to reduce free testosterone and increase sex hormone binding globulin (SHBG)
- *Lactating women:* progestin-only methods preferable to COCs in exclusively breast-feeding women. COCs may be initiated when baby's diet supplemented by other sources of nutrition or after lactation well established (if patient prefers COCs)
- *Hypercholesterolemia:* Selection of pill depends on type of dyslipidemia:
  - Elevated LDL or low HDL: consider estrogenic pill (high estrogen/progestin ratio) with low androgenicity
  - Elevated triglycerides: Some clinicians recommend not prescribing COCs if triglycerides > 350 because expect COCs to increase triglycerides by 30%.

- *Hepatic enzyme-inducing agents (e.g. anticonvulsants except valproic acid):* Options include:
  - Prescribe high-dose COC (containing 50 µg EE)
  - Prescribe 30-35 µg pill with reduced pill-free interval (first-day start, bicycling with first day start, or continuous use)
  - Prescribe 35 µg pill and use backup for 3 cycles. If no breakthrough bleeding by third cycle, discontinue backup method. If she has breakthrough bleeding, increase hormone levels or continue use of backup method (least reliable technique)
- *Antibiotic use:* Concern that without intestinal flora to unconjugate the hormonal compounds produced by first hepatic processing, subsequent reabsorption of estrogen and progestin would not be possible. However, recent research suggests <u>no</u> significant difference in circulating serum levels of hormones when women used broad-spectrum antibiotics. Class OC labeling warns about potential antibiotic interaction. For more complete discussion go to: www.managingcontraception.com/questions_new/oral/g_a_ or _06-12.html. If patient ←
  has other risk factor (vomiting, diarrhea, forgetfulness) or prefers, suggest back-up method for duration of antibiotic use

INSTRUCTIONS FOR PATIENT: Periodic "breaks" from pills are NOT recommended!
- Key to successful pill use is a well-informed patient. Provide new-start patients with:
  - Clear instructions on pill initiation, preferably written and in her native language ←
    and culturally sensitive
  - Concrete planning for COC use: where to store packet, how to remember to take, where and how she will obtain refills
  - Explanation about possible transitional side effects (spotting, breast tenderness, headaches, etc.) and encouragement to return should any become troublesome (see PROBLEM MANAGEMENT). Also highlight noncontraceptive benefits
  - Warning about serious complications (see ACHES, Figure 27.1 below & A-21)
- Backup method: ensure patient has and knows how to use method if she needs to use one for interim protection, back-up, or as an alternate method if she ever discontinues COC use
- Have patient return in 3 months for BP check and follow-up of any transition issues. Subsequently, only annual routine gynecologic exams are needed for low-risk patients

FOLLOW-UP CHECKLIST AT EACH RETURN VISIT:
NOTE: it is better to ask specific questions than to ask "Are you having any problems?"
- Are you having any symptoms of pregnancy?
- Are you having any changes in your periods? (see Figure 27.3 on page 109)
- Are you having any problems remembering to take your pills? (see PROBLEM MANAGEMENT)
- Are you having any breast tenderness, upset stomach, increased acne, mood changes, changes in your sex life, weight changes, headaches or other health problems?
- What medications are you taking?
- How much do you smoke?
- Are you having any of the ACHES problems?

Figure 27.1 PILL WARNING SIGNALS (ACHES) see also Appendix (A-21)

ACHES: A way to remember pill danger signals	
A	Abdominal pain? Yellow skin or eyes?
C	Chest pain?
H	Headaches that are severe?
E	Eye problems: blurred vision or loss of vision?
S	Severe leg pain or swelling (in the calf or thigh)?

PROBLEM MANAGEMENT

Nausea/vomiting: **Rule out pregnancy, reassure that nausea usually improves**

- Suggest taking pills at night (evening meal or bedtime) to allow patient to sleep through high serum levels of hormones. Suggest taking pills with morning meal if ← experiencing bothersome nausea during the night
- If patient vomits within one hour of taking pill, suggest antiemetic prior to taking replacement pill
- If nausea consistently occurs ≤ 2 hours after taking pill and is associated with headache and/or dizziness, consider hypoglycemia
- Abdominal pain should make you think of following problems that could be related to COC use: thrombosis of major intra-abdominal vessels, gallstones, pancreatis, liver adenoma, Crohn's disease or porphyria

Spotting and/or breakthrough bleeding: (see Figure 27.3, p. 109)

Missed one pill: **Instruct patient to take missed pill ASAP and take next pill as usual**

- Offer emergency contraceptive pills (ECPs), especially if missed pill is at beginning of pack. Start COCs next day after last EC dose

Missed two pills:

- Instruct patient to take one of the forgotten pills every 12 hours until she gets caught up, then continue rest of pack. Suggest long-acting antiemetic one hour before second pill if drowsiness is not a problem. Backup contraception recommended for 7 days
- Alternatively, offer ECPs, especially if patient is early in cycle and restart next day

Missed more than two pills: **Offer ECPs**

- If patient declines ECPs, instruct patient to skip missed pills and complete rest of pills in pack, but to use barrier method with each act of intercourse until her next menses. Advise patient that pills may not provide protection, but will help control her cycle

If patient uses ECPs: **Advise patient to skip the missed COCs in her pack**

- Instruct patient to resume taking pills in pack the next day after she finishes ECPs

Missed menses on COCs:

- Offer pregnancy test, especially if she missed any pills in last cycle or if she has any symptoms of pregnancy
- Offer emergency contraception if any recent unprotected intercourse
- Advise patient that there are no adverse clinical impacts of amenorrhea from COCs
- If patient prefers monthly menses, consider switching to formulation with higher estrogen or lower progestin
- Otherwise, have her continue her COCs on usual schedule

New onset or significant worsening of headaches on COCs: (see Figure 27.4, p. 110)

Hot flashes on placebo-pill week

- Suggest first-day start each cycle with any formulation or continuous use with monophasic pills
- Offer low-dose of transdermal or oral estrogen during placebo-pill week

MAKING THE TRANSITION FROM COCs TO HORMONE REPLACEMENT THERAPY: (See Figure 27.5, p. 111)

FERTILITY AFTER USE

- Rapid return to fertility: Average delay in ovulation 1-2 weeks. Rarely, post-pill amenorrhea may persist for up to 6 months. Post-pill amenorrhea is usually in women with history of ← very irregular menses prior to initiating COCs
- Women should initiate another method immediately after discontinuing COCs
- Women should be advised that their pattern of menses prior to starting pills (frequency, duration, flow, dysmenorrhea) tends to return once they stop COCs

Table 27.1 Starting Combined Oral Contraceptives*

CONDITION BEFORE STARTING	WHEN TO START COCs?
Starting (restarting) COCs in menstruating women	• First day of next menses or • First Sunday after next menses begins • Immediately, if pregnancy excluded start with pill appropriate for her cycle day**
Postpartum and breast-feeding	Wait at least until the baby is receiving significant nutritional supplement (AAP) After stopping breast-feeding, if amenorrheic (must be 21 days or more postpartum) • Immediately*** or • Next Sunday***
Postpartum and not breast-feeding (after pregnancy of 24 or more weeks)	• Wait 3-4 weeks after delivery to allow hypercoagulable state of pregnancy to abate
After first or second trimester (≤ 24 weeks) pregnancy loss or termination	• Immediately or • Next Sunday**
Switching from POPs or from other COCs to a COC	• At end of pack of pills or • Next Sunday** or • Immediately
After Norplant or IUD removal	• Immediately or • Next Sunday**
After DMPA	• Last day of efficacy (91 days) or • Earlier (immediately or next Sunday)
Secondary amenorrhea (POP-induced or DMPA- induced or other cause), when pregnancy is excluded	• Immediately** or • Next Sunday**
After taking ECPs	• Day after ECP** or • First day of next menses or • Sunday of next menses**

*. Adapted from Guillebaud J. Contraception Today, 3rd ed. London: Martin Dunitz Ltd., 1997
** Back-up method needed until 7 days after starting COCs
*** Back-up method needed until 7 days after starting COCs only if more than 6 months postpartum

---

➤➤ CASE: A 20 year-old university student is confused. In the middle of a package of pills she misses a pill and takes Lo-Ovral 4 tabs followed by 4 more tabs in 12 hours as ECPs. She wonders if she should wait until her next period to start back on her regular pill. Her physician suggests starting back on her ongoing pills the day after her second dose of ECPs and to use condoms for the next 7 days as a backup method of birth control.

NOTE: As this case suggests, there are many instances when a clinician may start pills other than on the first day of the next menstrual period or the first Sunday after the next period begins.

Figure 27.2

CHOOSING A PILL

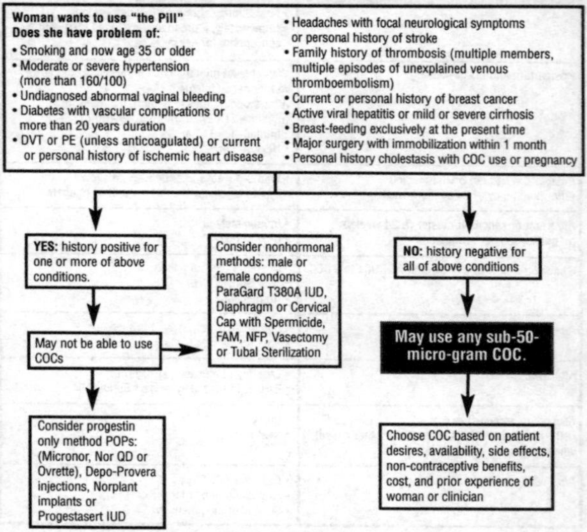

Woman wants to use "the Pill"
Does she have problem of:
- Smoking and now age 35 or older
- Moderate or severe hypertension (more than 160/100)
- Undiagnosed abnormal vaginal bleeding
- Diabetes with vascular complications or more than 20 years duration
- DVT or PE (unless anticoagulated) or current or personal history of ischemic heart disease

- Headaches with focal neurological symptoms or personal history of stroke
- Family history of thrombosis (multiple members, multiple episodes of unexplained venous thromboembolism)
- Current or personal history of breast cancer
- Active viral hepatitis or mild or severe cirrhosis
- Breast-feeding exclusively at the present time
- Major surgery with immobilization within 1 month
- Personal history cholestasis with COC use or pregnancy

| **YES:** history positive for one or more of above conditions | Consider nonhormonal methods: male or female condoms, ParaGard T380A IUD, Diaphragm or Cervical Cap with Spermicide, FAM, NFP, Vasectomy or Tubal Sterilization | **NO:** history negative for all of above conditions |

May not be able to use COCs

May use any sub-50-micro-gram COC.

Consider progestin only method POPs: (Micronor, Nor QD or Ovrette), Depo-Provera injections, Norplant implants or Progestasert IUD

Choose COC based on patient desires, availability, side effects, non-contraceptive benefits, cost, and prior experience of woman or clinician

- The World Health Organization and the Food and Drug Administration both recommend using the lowest dose pill that is effective. All combined pills with less than 50 μg of estrogen are effective and safe.
- There are no studies demonstrating a decreased risk for deep vein thrombosis (DVT) in women on 20-μg pills. Data on higher dose pills have demonstrated that the less the estrogen dose, the lower the risk for DVT.
- All COCs lower free testosterone. In the US, only Ortho Tri-Cyclen has FDA labeling indicating it as a treatment of moderate acne vulgaris, based on results of two randomized, placebo controlled trials. Other formulations are under study. Class labeling in Canada for all combined pills states that use of pills may improve acne. In Canada only, Tri-Cyclen has "treatment of moderate acne vulgaris" as an indication for use
- To minimize discontinuation due to spotting and breakthrough bleeding, warn women in advance, reassure that spotting and breakthrough bleeding become better over time. (See Figure 27.3, p. 109)
- To attain the most favorable lipid profile, consider norgestimate, desogestrel pill or low dose norethindrone acetate, or lowest dose norethindrone (Ovcon-35) or ethnodial diacetate (Demulen 1/35 or Zovia 35). No clinical benefits have been demonstrated to be attributable to difference in lipids caused by these pills. Estrogen has a beneficial effect on the walls of blood vessels. All currently available COCs raise triglycerides.

108

Figure 27.3

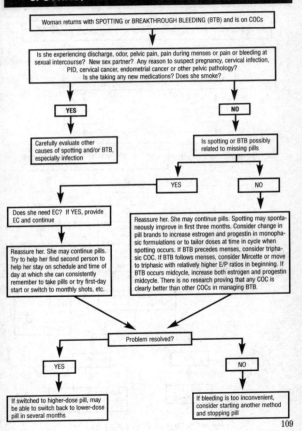

SPOTTING/BREAKTHROUGH BLEEDING ON COCs

Woman returns with SPOTTING or BREAKTHROUGH BLEEDING (BTB) and is on COCs

Is she experiencing discharge, odor, pelvic pain, pain during menses or pain or bleeding at sexual intercourse? New sex partner? Any reason to suspect pregnancy, cervical infection, PID, cervical cancer, endometrial cancer or other pelvic pathology?
Is she taking any new medications? Does she smoke?

YES

Carefully evaluate other causes of spotting and/or BTB, especially infection

NO

Is spotting or BTB possibly related to missing pills

YES

Does she need EC? If YES, provide EC and continue

Reassure her. She may continue pills. Try to help her find second person to help her stay on schedule and time of day at which she can consistently remember to take pills or try first-day start or switch to monthly shots, etc.

NO

Reassure her. She may continue pills. Spotting may spontaneously improve in first three months. Consider change in pill brands to increase estrogen and progestin in monophasic formulations or to tailor doses at time in cycle when spotting occurs. If BTB precedes menses, consider triphasic COC. If BTB follows menses, consider Mircette or move to triphasic with relatively higher E/P ratios in beginning. If BTB occurs midcycle, increase both estrogen and progestin midcycle. There is no research proving that any COC is clearly better than other COCs in managing BTB.

Problem resolved?

YES

If switched to higher-dose pill, may be able to switch back to lower-dose pill in several months

NO

If bleeding is too inconvenient, consider starting another method and stopping pill

Figure 27.4

NEW ONSET OR WORSENING HEADACHES IN COC USERS

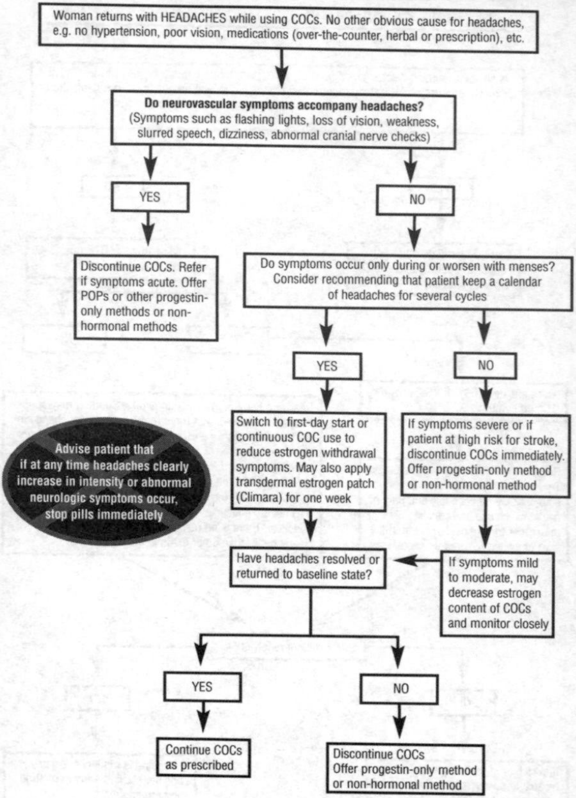

Woman returns with HEADACHES while using COCs. No other obvious cause for headaches, e.g. no hypertension, poor vision, medications (over-the-counter, herbal or prescription), etc.

↓

Do neurovascular symptoms accompany headaches?
(Symptoms such as flashing lights, loss of vision, weakness, slurred speech, dizziness, abnormal cranial nerve checks)

YES → Discontinue COCs. Refer if symptoms acute. Offer POPs or other progestin-only methods or non-hormonal methods.

NO → Do symptoms occur only during or worsen with menses? Consider recommending that patient keep a calendar of headaches for several cycles

YES → Switch to first-day start or continuous COC use to reduce estrogen withdrawal symptoms. May also apply transdermal estrogen patch (Climara) for one week

NO → If symptoms severe or if patient at high risk for stroke, discontinue COCs immediately. Offer progestin-only method or non-hormonal method

If symptoms mild to moderate, may decrease estrogen content of COCs and monitor closely

Advise patient that if at any time headaches clearly increase in intensity or abnormal neurologic symptoms occur, stop pills immediately

Have headaches resolved or returned to baseline state?

YES → Continue COCs as prescribed

NO → Discontinue COCs. Offer progestin-only method or non-hormonal method

Figure 27.5

MAKING THE TRANSITION FROM COCs TO HORMONE REPLACEMENT THERAPY (HRT)

The transition from COCs to HRT is accomplished in a number of ways. Some reviewers of this algorithm switch to a 20-mcg pill if the patient is going to use COCs into the early 50s.

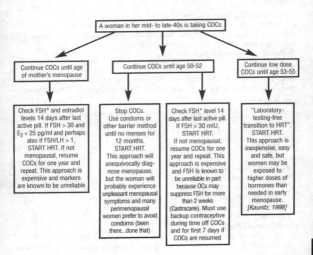

A woman in her mid- to late-40s is taking COCs

Continue COCs until age of mother's menopause

Check FSH* and estradiol levels 14 days after last active pill. If FSH > 30 and E₂ < 25 pg/ml and perhaps also if FSH/LH > 1, START HRT. If not menopausal, resume COCs for one year and repeat. This approach is expensive and markers are known to be unreliable.

Continue COCs until age 50-52

Stop COCs. Use condoms or other barrier method until no menses for 12 months. START HRT. This approach will unequivocally diagnose menopause, but the woman will probably experience unpleasant menopausal symptoms and many perimenopausal women prefer to avoid condoms (been there...done that)

Check FSH* level 14 days after last active pill. If FSH > 30 mIU, START HRT. If not menopausal, resume COCs for one year and repeat. This approach is expensive and FSH is known to be unreliable in part because OCs may suppress FSH for more than 2 weeks (Castracane). Must use backup contraception during time off COCs and for first 7 days if COCs are resumed

Continue low dose COCs until age 53-55

"Laboratory-testing-free transition to HRT". START HRT. This approach is inexpensive, easy and safe, but women may be exposed to higher doses of hormones than needed in early menopause. *[Kaunitz, 1998]*

*FSH and LH testing are problematic. Lab testing only indicates the here and now - a perimenopausal woman can seem to be menopausal according to lab tests but ovulate 2 months later. ◄

DESCRIPTION

1 cc of a crystalline suspension of 150 mg depot medroxyprogesterone acetate injected intramuscularly into the deltoid or gluteus maximus muscle every 11-13 weeks. For more information call 1-800-253-8600 ext 38244

EFFECTIVENESS *(Trussell J, Contraceptive Technology, 1998)*

• Approved labeling indicates each injection effective for up to 13 weeks

Perfect use failure rate in first year: less than 0.3% (fewer than 3 in every 1000 users will become pregnant during the first year) (See Table 13.2, p. 36)

Typical use failure rate in first year: 0.3%

MECHANISMS

Suppresses ovulation by inhibiting LH surge, thickens cervical mucus to block sperm entry into female upper reproductive tract, slows tubal and endometrial mobility, and may alter endometrium

COST in 1995

Setting	Managed care	Public provider
Drug	$30/13 weeks	$30/13 weeks
Office visit	$38/13 weeks	$16.56/13 weeks

ADVANTAGES

Menstrual:

• Decreased menstrual blood loss
• After 1 year of use, 50% of women achieve amenorrhea; 80% achieve amenorrhea in 5 years
• Decreased menstrual cramps, pain and ovulation pain
• Possible improvement in endometriosis
• Prevents hemorrhagic corpus luteum cysts

Sexual/psychological:

• Intercourse may be more pleasurable without worry of pregnancy
• Convenient: permits spontaneous sexual activity; requires no action at time of intercourse

Cancers, tumors, and masses:

• Significant reduction in risk of endometrial cancer
• Possible reduction in risk of ovarian cancer

Benefits for women with medical problems:

• Suppresses ovulation, bleeding and menstrual blood loss in anticoagulated women and women with bleeding diathesis
• Reduces acute sickle cell crises by 70%
• Best method for women taking anticonvulsant medications; may decrease seizures
• Amenorrhea and prolonged effective contraception may be very important for severely developmentally or physically disabled women
• Decreases anemia
• Possible improvement of endometriosis

Other:
- Prevents ectopic pregnancies
- Decreases risk of PID
- Convenient: single injection provides at least 13 weeks protection
- Forgiving: effective in many women for more than 13 weeks
- Less user-dependent than POPs, COCs
- Good option for women who can not use estrogen (see CANDIDATES FOR USE)
- Private: no visible clue that patient is using; no one else needs to know
- May be used by nursing mothers

DISADVANTAGES

Menstrual:
- Irregular menses during first several months: many women experience unpredictable spotting and bleeding, occasionally blood loss reported to be heavy but unlikely to cause anemia. After 6-12 months, amenorrhea more likely

Sexual/psychological:
- Spotting and bleeding may interfere with sexual activity
- Amenorrhea may raise fears of pregnancy or "unclean womb" (not clinically correct)
- Hypoestrogenism can (infrequently) cause dyspareunia, hot flashes or decreased libido
- Possible increase in depression, anxiety, irritation, PMS, fatigue or other mood changes, but often DMPA reduces risk of these disorders
- Fear of needles may make this an unacceptable choice

Cancers, tumors, and masses: None

Other:
- No protection against STIs: must use condoms if at risk
- Must return every 11-13 weeks for injection
- Long acting: not reversible once injected
- Slow to return to fertility: average 10 months from last injection
- Occasionally, hypoestrogenism ($E_2 < 25$) may develop as a result of FSH suppression. Vasomotor symptoms and potential for decreased bone mineral density if used for prolonged period without opportunity for recovery prior to menopause
- Severe headaches may occur
- Acne, hirsutism may develop
- Possible increase in diabetes risk with breast-feeding gestational diabetes woman first year postpartum [Kjos 1999]
- Metabolic impacts: glucose (slight rise), LDL (slight rise or neutral), HDL (may decrease)
- Other hormone-related symptoms: breast tenderness, bloating, hair loss, weight gain/ weight loss, etc.
- See COMPLICATIONS below

COMPLICATIONS
- Progressive significant weight gain
- Severe depression (rare) (average MMPI does not change in women on DMPA)
- Severe allergic reaction, including anaphylaxis (very rare). May consider having women wait in or near office for 20 minutes after injection. (Reviewers disagree about this recommendation, especially for previous DMPA users)

CANDIDATES FOR USE

- Women who want intermediate-to-long-term contraception and can return every 11-13 weeks
- Especially appropriate for:
  - Women who want privacy, convenience, and high efficacy
  - Women who want or need to avoid estrogen:
    - Women with personal history of thrombosis (WHO: 2) or strong family history of venous thromboembolism (WHO: 1)
    - Recently postpartum women (WHO: 1)
    - Women who are exclusively breast-feeding beyond 6 weeks postpartum (WHO: 1). There is debate about use of DMPA in breastfeeding women less than 6 weeks PP
    - Smokers over age 35 (WHO: 1)
    - Women who had or fear chloasma, vomiting, migraine headaches, hypertriglyceridemia, or other estrogen-related side effects
  - Women who use drugs which affect liver clearance (except aminoglutethimide)
  - Women with anemia, fibroids, seizure disorder (WHO 1), sickle cell disease (WHO: 1), endometriosis, hypertriglyceridemia (WHO: 2), systemic lupus erythematosus or coagulation disorder (hyper- or hypo-coagulation)

Adolescent women – positive features: (WHO: 2)

- Extremely effective with long carry-over if patient returns late for reinjection
- Privacy and confidentiality possible
- Decreases menstrual cramps and pain

Adolescent women – special issues:

- For some teens (especially those who have experienced a pregnancy) may be only ⟵ acceptable method that offers high efficacy
- May be associated with significant weight gain, acne, complexion changes
- Requires periodic reinjections
- Long-term impact on bone mineralization is not known. Studies suggest mineralization suppressed during teen growth period. May be reversible (studies ongoing). Protocol: see **managingcontraception.com**
- No STI protection: Must use condoms if at risk

PRESCRIBING PRECAUTIONS

- Pregnancy
- Undiagnosed abnormal vaginal bleeding
- Unable to tolerate injections
- History of breast cancer, MI or stroke
- Current venous thromboembolism (unless anticoagulated)
- Liver dysfunction
- Known hypersensitivity to Depo-Provera

DRUG INTERACTIONS: Aminoglutethimide reduces DMPA efficacy

MEDICAL ELIGIBILITY CHECKLIST

Ask the client the questions below. If she answers NO to ALL the questions, then she CAN use DMPA if she wants. If she answers YES to a question below, follow the instructions

1. Do you think you are pregnant?

☐ No ☐ Yes   Assess if pregnant. If she might be pregnant, give her condoms or spermicide to use until reasonably sure that she is not pregnant. Then she can start DMPA

2. Do you plan to become pregnant in the next year?

☐ No ☐ Yes   Use another method with less delay in return of fertility

3. Do you have serious medical problems such as heart attack (WHO: 3), severe chest pain, or uncontrolled high blood pressure (WHO: 2 or 3)? Have you ever had such problems? (See page A-3)

☐ No ☐ Yes   In general, do not provide DMPA if she reports heart attack, stroke, heart disease due to blocked arteries, severe high blood pressure, diabetes for more than 20 years, or damage to vision, kidneys, or nervous system caused by diabetes. Help her choose another effective method. All the above conditions receive a "3" in the 2001 WHO Medical Eligibility Criteria (see Appendix pages A-2 and A-3)

4. Do you have or have you ever had breast cancer (WHO: 3 or 4)? (See page A-5)

☐ No ☐ Yes   Do not provide DMPA. Help her choose a method without hormones

5. Do you have jaundice, cirrhosis of the liver, a liver infection or tumor? (Are her eyes or skin unusually yellow?) (See page A-5)

☐ No ☐ Yes   Perform physical exam or refer. If she has serious liver disease (jaundice, painful or enlarged liver, viral hepatitis, liver tumor), do not provide DMPA. Refer for care. Help her choose a method without hormones

6. Do you have vaginal bleeding that is unusual for you? (See page A-4)

☐ No ☐ Yes   If she is not pregnant but has unexplained vaginal bleeding that suggest an underlying medical condition, assess and treat any underlying condition as appropriate, or refer. Provide DMPA based on findings

7. For patients who delivered < than 1 year ago. Did you have diabetes (See p. A-6) with this pregnancy and do you plan to breast-feed (See p. A-2)?

☐ No ☐ Yes   Advise patient there may be some increased risk of developing glucose intolerance or frank diabetes the first year if she has no periods on DMPA. If there is no other good method for her, she may use Depo-Provera

INITIATING METHOD (see Figure 28.1)

Cycling women:
- Preferred start time is during first 5 days from the start of menses
- Alternative: may inject anytime in the cycle when she is not pregnant, but have patient use back-up method for 7 days after injection (off-label).

Postpartum women: May give first injection prior to hospital discharge. Special considerations:
- After severe obstetrical blood loss, delay injection until lochia stops
- If woman has history or high risk for severe postpartum depression, delay injection 4-6 weeks
- Breast-feeding women: If mother's nutrition is adequate, start DMPA immediately. Otherwise, wait 4-6 weeks

Women who have spontaneous or therapeutic abortion: May initiate immediately.

Women switching methods:
- May start anytime patient is known not to be pregnant
- If switching from non-hormonal method, offer same options as cycling women

INSTRUCTIONS FOR PATIENT
- Do not massage area where shot was given for first few hours
- Expect irregular bleeding/spotting in beginning. Usually decreases over time
- Return at any time spotting or bleeding is bothersome. Treatments available that may make bleeding pattern more tolerable
- After 6-12 months, most women have little or no bleeding. It is not harmful or dangerous if you do not have periods while you use DMPA
- Weight change is common. More women gain weight than lose weight with DMPA. Watch what you eat (even if you feel hungrier) and exercise

> ### WEIGHT GAIN: A TEACHABLE MOMENT
>
> When you see a patient who is very heavy or has gained some weight that disturbs her, you have a teachable moment. BE PREPARED FOR THAT TEACHABLE MOMENT. Here are several suggestions that take but a minute to share.
>
> *Helping someone to lose weight in 60 seconds!*
>
> 1. Eat less (small, frequent meals helps some to lose weight)
> 2. Exercise more
> 3. Find patterns of eating and exercising that you enjoy! You won't do them for long unless you enjoy the process.
> 4. Call Overeaters Anonymous (OA), a free source of love and caring. OA works!
> 5. Drink 10 glasses of water daily

- Be sure to take 1000 mg (women over age 25) to 1300 mg (adolescent women) calcium every day to build your bones. Get exercise 3 times a week (good for general health)
- Return in 11-13 weeks for your next injection. Use abstinence after 13 weeks. Rush in if it has been more than 13 weeks
- Have condoms and EC ready to use if you are ever late coming for your re-injection

- Pregnancy is very rare, but return for care promptly if you develop any pregnancy symptoms
- Serious complications with Depo-Provera are rare, but return if you have worsening severe headaches; heavy bleeding; depression; severe lower abdominal pain; problems at the shot site (pus, pain or bleeding)

FOLLOW-UP
- What is happening to your menstrual periods?
- Did you have pain at the injection site after previous injection?
- Have you felt depressed or had major mood changes?
- Have you gained 5 pounds or more? (See WEIGHT GAIN, A TEACHABLE MOMENT, p. 116)
- Do you have any increase in your headaches?
- Have you had severe lower abdominal pain, nausea or vomiting?
- Have you had the feeling that you may be pregnant?
- Have you had any pain with intercourse or an unusual vaginal discharge?
- Did you have any problems returning on time for this injection?
- When do you plan to become pregnant?

PROBLEM MANAGEMENT
Administration problems
Allergic reaction or vasovagal reaction:
In acute setting, provide support as needed. Benadryl may reduce pruritus and swelling. Oxygen and other resuscitation may be needed for severe reactions (extremely rare). Most allergic manifestations subside in 1 week or so. Refer if symptoms severe or do not improve appropriately. Avoid future injections.

Vaginal dryness (dyspareunia) or atrophic vaginitis:
May be due to hypoestrogenism. Consider measuring E_2 levels and giving physiologic replacement dose of estrogen, if needed. Consider estrogen vaginal cream ring, tablets ← or systemic estrogen (tablets or patch) supplementation. Dyspareunia may be relieved with lubricant.

Pain or infection at injection site:
Offer anti-inflammatory medications. Rule out infection or needle damage to nerve, etc. Provide appropriate antibiotics if infected. Avoid massaging area for first several hours after injection.

Patient returns late (>13 weeks) for reinjection: See Figure 28.1 on page 119

Switching to another method (eg OCs, IUD, etc) from DMPA:
Initiate new method at any time convenient for patient, but preferred time would be near end of effectiveness of last DMPA injection (11-13 weeks) unless switching to OCs to control menstrual disorders on DMPA

Transitioning perimenopausal women: See Figure 28.2 on page 120

Problems with usage:
Weight gain:
Advise patient to watch her calorie intake carefully (DMPA may make her feel hungry) and to increase exercise. Discontinue method if weight gain is excessive or unacceptable

Heavy bleeding:
- Rule out pregnancy, cervical infection, and cervical cancer
- Rule out anemia - recommend iron rich foods and/or supplements
- May treat with NSAIDs or low dose estrogen supplements:
  - Ibuprofen 800 mg orally every 8 hours for 3 days
  - Conjugated equine estrogen (.625, 1.25, or 2.5 mg) orally up to four times per day for 4-6 days (may not be as effective as with Norplant)
  - Estrogenic COCs for 1-2 months
  - Note: Physiologic estrogen replacement may be continued indefinitely with DMPA use. COCs should be limited to next injection or two. NSAIDs may be used periodically with limit of 2400 mg of ibuprofen per 24 hour period. Avoid NSAIDs in patients with GI disorder or asthma
- May need to switch to another method; consider COCs or Lunelle

Irregular bleeding and spotting:
Reassure that irregular spotting and bleeding is to be expected in first several months.
May use same therapies as outlined in heavy bleeding section above

Amenorrhea:
Reassure patient that this is not a medical problem. Do pregnancy test only if she has other symptoms. Switch method if patient desires menses (Consider Lunelle, the estrogen-progestin monthly injection) Keep in mind, even if DMPA patient switches to Lunelle or COCs, menses may not return for many months

Depression:
Reevaluate suicide potential and refer immediately, if indicated. Patient should avoid alcohol. Explain that DMPA usually does not worsen depression. Start antidepressant therapy, if needed. May discontinue DMPA if patient has any misgivings about continuing its use

FERTILITY AFTER USE
- Return to fertility is delayed but excellent after using DMPA
- Average of 9-10 months delay to conception after last injection. This delay does not increase with increased duration of use
- More than 90% of women become pregnant within 2 years of discontinuing DMPA
- Because anovulation may last for more than 1 year, women who know they will want to become pregnant within one year of cessation of use would be wise to consider another option
- Women who do not want to await spontaneous return of ovulation will require gonadotrophin therapy to induce ovulation. Gonadotrophins will not overcome effect of DMPA on cervical mucus

Figure 28.1 Initial Injection or Late Reinjection (more than 13 weeks since last injection) of DMPA or Switching From DMPA to COCs or Another Hormonal Method*

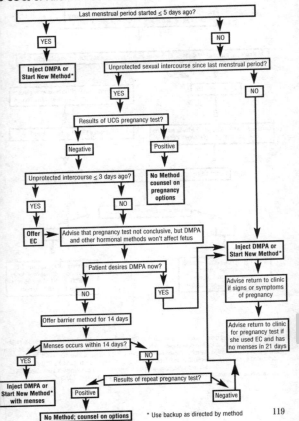

* Use backup as directed by method

Figure 28.2 Making Transition from DMPA in Perimenopausal Women

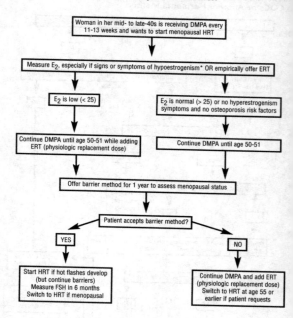

Woman in her mid- to late-40s is receiving DMPA every 11-13 weeks and wants to start menopausal HRT

↓

Measure E_2, especially if signs or symptoms of hypoestrogenism* OR empirically offer ERT

↓

E_2 is low (< 25)

E_2 is normal (> 25) or no hyperestrogenism symptoms and no osteoporosis risk factors

↓

Continue DMPA until age 50-51 while adding ERT (physiologic replacement dose)

Continue DMPA until age 50-51

↓

Offer barrier method for 1 year to assess menopausal status

↓

Patient accepts barrier method?

YES

NO

Start HRT if hot flashes develop (but continue barriers)
Measure FSH in 6 months
Switch to HRT if menopausal

Continue DMPA and add ERT (physiologic replacement dose)
Switch to HRT at age 55 or earlier if patient requests

* DMPA can suppress gonadotropins, so measuring FSH or LH is not informative of menopausal state. DMPA use decreases endogenous estrogen levels. Long-term DMPA users in their 40s may benefit from estrogen supplementation. Kaunitz supplements long-term DMPA users in their 40s with 1.25 mg of conjugated estrogen (or equivalent drug). Arbitrarily, at age 55, each woman can be switched to conventional HRT. This is easy and minimizes need for laboratory testing, addresses bone density issue, contraception, vasomotor concerns while maintaining amenorrhea. [Kaunitz, 1998]

DESCRIPTION: 0.5 cc suspension containing 25 mg medroxyprogesterone acetate and 5 mg estradiol cypionate injected intramuscularly into the deltoid or gluteus maximus muscle every 28 ± 5 days. Estradiol cypionate is metabolized to estradiol in the bloodstream. Brand names: Lunelle, Lunella, Cyclo-Provera, Cyclofem. More information: 1-800-253-8600 ext. 38244

EFFECTIVENESS (See Table 13.2, p. 36)
Perfect use failure rate in first year: 0.1-0.4/100 women (WHO data and U.S. trials)
Typical first year failure rate: Same

MECHANISMS: Same as COCs; primary mechanism is suppression of ovulation

COST: Price of drug expected to be similar to brand-name COCs. Price of administration of drug may vary. Public clinic price: $16.61; Direct order: $19.96; Average price when ← purchased at pharmacy: $24.95. Cost of medication plus injection in 4 physicians offices in Southeastern U.S. in April 2001: $35. Range of cost in physicians offices is from $32 to $45.

ADVANTAGES

Menstrual:
- Excellent cycle control after first few cycles
- Decreases ovulatory pain (Mittelschmerz); may decrease dysmenorrhea
- Prevents internal hemorrhage from ovulation in women with coagulation defects
- Prevents hemorrhagic corpus luteal cysts

Sexual/psychological:
- May enhance sexual enjoyment due to diminished fear of pregnancy
- Convenient: one injection provides up to 33 days protection. No disruption at time of intercourse; facilitates spontaneity

Cancers, tumors, and masses: No documented impacts, but probably similar to protective effects of COCs

Other:
- 10 day window of time (28 ± 5 days) over which injections may be given (flexibility!) ← In average woman, ovulation on Lunelle actually is suppressed for about 40 days which is more than 28 + 5 days
- Effectiveness, convenience, rapid reversibility, and privacy
- May diminish adverse effects on lipids seen with COCs
- May reduce risk of PID
- No clotting or cardiovascular complications in WHO studies ←

DISADVANTAGES

Menstrual:
- Approximately 6-8% of women discontinue because of menstrual irregularities
- Increased number of days of spotting/bleeding in first month of use. Then predictable pattern established which closely corresponds to patient's usual baseline pattern
- Amenorrhea in 1% (first cycle) to 4% (60th week) of cycles. In cycles 2-12, 15% ← of Lunelle users experienced a missed period

121

Sexual/physiological:
- Depression, anxiety, irritability, fatigue or other mood changes may develop (although not documented to occur at higher rates than COCs)
- Fear of needles may preclude use of this method

Cancers, tumors, and masses: No documented impact

Other:
- Must return each month for reinjection (every 28 ± 5 days); may be confused with the 13-week/3 month regimen called Depo-Provera. Pharmacia-Upjohn is developing a system to remind Lunelle users each month that their Lunelle injection is coming up; this will be done through e-mail
- Weight gain in one year (median values: 2-4 lbs. in women ≤ 150 lbs.; 2-6 lbs. in women > 150 lbs.)
- Not immediately reversible if side effects develop
- No protection against STIs. Must use condoms if at risk
- Mastalgia reported and other hormonal side effects

COMPLICATIONS: Somewhat similar to COCs (see pages 99-100). Less thrombophilic. There may be injection site problems

CANDIDATES FOR USE
- Women who are candidates for estrogen/progestin combined hormonal medication and who
  - Appreciate convenience of injections and desire more regular menses than women experience with DMPA
- Had difficulty remembering COCs or bleeding irregularities on DMPA or Norplant

Adolescents: private method, but requires monthly visits, which may be difficult

PRESCRIBING PRECAUTIONS: Similar to COCs (see p. 99-103 & Appendix, A-1–A-8)
- Known or suspected pregnancy
- Thrombophlebitis or thromboembolic disorder; History of DVT or VTE disorders
- Severe hypertension
- Cerebral vascular or coronary artery disease
- Diabetes with vascular involvement
- Undiagnosed abnormal vaginal bleeding
- Liver dysfunction or disease such as hepatic adenoma or carcinoma; history of cholestatic jaundice of pregnancy or jaundice with prior hormonal contraceptive use
- Valvular heart disease with complications
- Estrogen dependent neoplasm (except endometriosis)
- Headaches with focal neurologic symptoms
- Known hypersensitivity to ingredients
- Smoking over age 35

DRUG INTERACTIONS: Unknown, but may be similar to COCs (see p. 105)
- Aminoglutethimide may decrease serum MPA levels
- Anticoagulants, rifampin, griseofulvin

INITIATING METHOD
First injection is to be given in first 5 days after onset of menses
No backup method needed

INSTRUCTIONS FOR PATIENT
Expect first menses early (2-3 weeks after injection)
Return in 28 ± 5 days (23-33 days) for next injection
Reinjections are not timed by your menses but by the calendar
Each subsequent menses depends on timing of previous injection

FOLLOW-UP
Patient should return every 28 ± 5 days for reinjection
Questions similar to COC questions

PROBLEM MANAGEMENT: Similar to COCs (see p. 106-110)

FERTILITY AFTER USE:
Excellent return to baseline fertility: 2 month delay from last injection

CHAPTER 30

Contraceptive Implants: Norplant

www.popcouncil.org or www.wyeth.com/news ←

DESCRIPTION: 6 soft plastic (silastic) implants (34 mm in length and 2.4 mm in diameter) are inserted into the subcutaneous tissue beneath the skin of the medial aspect of a woman's non-dominant upper arm. Each implant is filled with 36 mg of levonorgestrel powder, which is slowly released through micropores in the implant to achieve an average plasma concentration of 0.30 ng/ml over 5 years. Since Norplant is no longer available, much of the information on this excellent method has been left out of this edition. Readers may obtain extensive information on Norplant from the 2000-2001 edition of *Managing Contraception*. As of April 21, 2001 it appears that Norplant will never be reintroduced in the U.S. ←

EFFECTIVENESS *[Trussell J. Contraceptive Technology 1998] (See Table 13.2, p. 36)*
• Product labeling indicates the system is effective for up to 5 years. Is effective for 7 years or more (see below)
Perfect use failure rate in first year: 0.05% (1 woman in 2,000)
Typical use failure rate in first year: 0.05%
Cumulative 7 year failure rate: 1.9% *[Contraception 61:187, 2000]* ←

MECHANISMS

The primary mechanism of action is to thicken the cervical mucus consistently throughout the cycle to block sperm penetration into the female upper reproductive tract and avoid fertilization. In the first 1-2 years of use when the circulating levonorgestrel levels are higher, ovulation is blocked in most women. However, by the fifth year of use, nearly 90% of users are routinely ovulating. The progesterone may create an inadequate luteal phase and a uterine environment that is suboptimal for implantation, but the clinical significance of these mechanisms has not been demonstrated.

COST: *See Managing Contraception 2000-2001*
• Norplant Foundation (1-800-760-9030) is available with funding to provide kits to indigent women not covered by other programs and to pay for simple or complicated removals in these women

ADVANTAGES
Menstrual:
• Decreases cumulative blood loss (mean monthly blood loss 25 cc vs 35 cc in controls)
• Decreases menstrual cramping and pain
• Decreases pain with ovulation in early years (Mittelschmerz)
Sexual/psychological:
• Reduction in pregnancy risk may make sexual activity more pleasurable
• Convenient: no action required at time of intercourse

ncers, tumors, and masses:
- May reduce risk of endometrial cancer and/or ovarian cancer. No data

hers:
- Highly effective and very cost effective over time
- Convenient: single insertion provides 5 years of protection
- Private: if correctly inserted deeply enough below skin, palpable but usually not obviously visible
- Decreases risk of PID
- Extremely low doses of progestin, no estrogen. Good option for women who can not use estrogen

olescent Issues:
- Adolescents have higher continuation rates with Norplant than with COCs or DMPA
- Lower pregnancy rates have been seen in teen mothers using Norplant compared to those using contraceptive pills

SADVANTAGES

nstrual:
- Irregular menses is very common during first year
- Usually in first year, women have more days of spotting and bleeding than nonusers, but have less total blood loss
- 20% have amenorrhea or oligomenorrhea
- After 6-12 months, many women re-establish predictable menstrual patterns, but significant minority persists with unpredictable patterns

xual/Psychological:
- Spotting and bleeding may interfere with sexual activities
- Possible increase in mood changes, depression, anxiety, irritability, fatigue
- Fear of needles (for injecting local anesthesia) or scalpel may make this an unacceptable choice
- Dislike of foreign bodies or hormones may preclude selection of this method

ncers, tumors or masses:
- Ovarian enlargement due to less suppression of FSH may lead to persistent ovarian follicles. Most follicular cysts regress spontaneously; watchful waiting is treatment for asymptomatic women

hers:
- Offers no protection against STIs. Must use condoms if at risk
- Insertion and removal require special procedure by trained medical personnel. Patient unable to discontinue method by herself
- Weight changes reported. Over half of women gain weight; about 20% lose weight. However, average 5-year weight gain similar to women not using Norplant
- Other hormonally-related side effects: breast tenderness, headaches, bloating, acne, vaginal discharge, hair growth, scalp hair loss, skin discoloration over implants, etc.
- Insertion/removal related issues: high initial cost, possible infection or scarring, expulsion, nerve or muscle damage (exceedingly rare), bruising and/or pain after procedure.

OMPLICATIONS: *See Managing Contraception 2000-2001*

ANDIDATES FOR USE: *See Managing Contraception 2000-2001*

RESCRIBING PRECAUTIONS: *See Managing Contraception 2000-2001*

MEDICAL ELIGIBILITY CHECKLIST: *See Managing Contraception 2000-2001*

INITIATING METHOD: *See Managing Contraception 2000-2001*

PRACTICAL TIPS ON PROPER NORPLANT INSERTION:
See Managing Contraception 2000-2001

INSTRUCTIONS FOR PATIENT: *See Managing Contraception 2000-2001*
- If you move and want implants removed, you may call the Norplant Foundation
  for names of clinicians who will remove implants and to get help with finances if needed.
  The number to call is 1-800-760-9030

FOLLOW-UP: *See Managing Contraception 2000-2001*

PROBLEM MANAGEMENT: *See Managing Contraception 2000-2001*

PRACTICAL TIPS ON PROPER NORPLANT REMOVAL
*Learning proper removal techniques requires formal training under direct
supervision. The tips that follow are brief reminders only:*
- Wyeth-Ayerst and Norplant Foundation provide a video on Norplant removal that is
  essential for clinicians to view prior to first Norplant removals.
- Use arm model to practice removal
- Identify both proximal and distal ends of each implant. Mark both ends
- Place anesthesia at the site of incision and beneath the distal one third to one half of each
  implant. Add NaHCO$_3$ to lidocaine to decrease stinging. Initially, inject approximately 3
  of 1% lidocaine. Have an additional 3-5 cc ready to provide additional anesthesia if needed.
  Alternatively, the proximal field block infusion may be very helpful (Figure 30.2)
- Three major techniques have been developed for implant removal. Learn all three to use
  in different situations. In each case, the goal is to isolate each implant in turn, incise
  through its surrounding fibrous sheath and remove only the implant.
  1. *Standard technique:* (see figure 30.5) Horizontal incision at base of implants. Dissect
     beneath tips to create plane. Grasp each implant with curved forceps and bring to
     incision. Incise through the fibrous sheath and grasp the implant with straight clamp
     and remove it (average removal time for 6 capsules is 20 minutes)

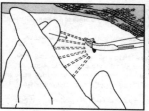

**Figure 30.5: Use of hemostat to
remove implant while clinician's
finger pushes implant towards
incision***

*Hatcher RA. Depo-Provera, Norplant, and
progestin-only pills (minipills). In: Hatcher
RA, et al. *Contraceptive Technology*. 17th e
New York: Ardent Media, 1998.

2. *Instrument-less (digital extrusion) technique:* Works well for superficial implants with tips all converging to same point. Infuse area at base with 0.1 cc local anesthesia. Cut directly down to implant and squeeze through tiny incision. Manipulate subsequent implants through same incision. (Learning curve is same as Standard technique. Patient satisfaction is very high)

3. *"Norgrasp" or Modified-U technique:* (see figure 30.6) Make vertical incision and create plane laterally beneath implants. Grasp each implant in turn with modified no-scalpel vasectomy clamp (Norgrasp clamp). Incise fibrous sheath and remove implants. (Average removal time 6.6 minutes. Quick learning curve)

Figure 30.6: U-technique for Norplant removal*

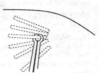

*Hatcher RA. Depo-provera, Norplant, and progestin-only pills (minipills). In: Hatcher RA, et al *Contraceptive Technology.* 17th ed. New York: Ardent Media, 1998:489

- Show patient all 6 implants
- Close incision with Steri-strips and pressure bandage
- Review post procedure instructions with patient

FERTILITY AFTER USE

- Return to baseline fertility is rapid and complete
- Levonorgestrel disappears from the circulation within 2 days

CHAPTER 31

Implanon: The Single Etonogestrel Implant

DESCRIPTION: Now available in the Netherlands, UK, Sweden, Germany, Belgium, Finland, Switzerland, Denmark and Austria. Coming soon to U.S. ◄
Single implant is 4-cm long and 2 mm in diameter (5 mm longer than one Norplant implant), with a membrane of ethylene vinyl acetate copolymer and with a core of 68 mg of etonogestrel (the new name for 3-ketodesogestrel). Progestin released at rate of 60 µg per day for effective life of 3 years. Implant is placed under the skin of upper arm with a disposable, preloaded inserter.

EFFECTIVENESS: Similar to Norplant, with effective life of 3 years. (0% pregnancy in first 70,000 cycles studied)

MECHANISM
- Within 24 hours of insertion thick cervical mucus prevents normal sperm transport
- Inhibition of ovulation (far greater than with Norplant implants) ◄
- Atrophic endometrium: inadequate development of secretory endometrium

COST: Not determined

ADVANTAGES
Menstrual: Decreased menstrual and ovulatory cramping or pain
Sexual/psychological:
- Sexual intercourse may be more pleasurable because fear of pregnancy is reduced
- Applied at time independent of sexual intercourse—allows spontaneity
Cancers/tumors and masses: None
Other:
- High continuation rate in clinical trials. Cyclic headaches may improve
- Single implant is easier and faster to insert and remove ◄

DISADVANTAGES
Menstrual:
- Irregular menstrual bleeding not uncommon initially
- Amenorrhea in 1/5 of users with time
Sexual/psychological:
- Irregular bleeding may inhibit sexual intercourse
- Insertion and removal require procedures, which may preclude use
Cancers/tumors and masses: None
Other:
- No STI protection
- Hormonal side effects: headache is most common

COMPLICATIONS (see Norplant) Removal complications much less frequent

PRESCRIBING PRECAUTIONS, CANDIDATES FOR USE, MEDICAL ELIGIBILITY CHECKLIST, INITIATING METHOD (see Norplant p. 123) (details - next edition!)

INSTRUCTIONS FOR PATIENT: Irregular bleeding is to be expected. If your pattern of bleeding is unacceptable, come back because there are several things that may be done to make your bleeding pattern more acceptable. Amenorrhea more likely than with Norplant, but less likely than with DMPA

FOLLOW-UP, PROBLEM MANAGEMENT (see Norplant p. 127, 128) (details - next edition!)

FERTILITY AFTER USING: Return to baseline fertility is rapid and complete; 94% ovulate within
month of removal

DESCRIPTION

Surgery to interrupt the fallopian tubes to prevent pregnancy. In 1995, 24% of married women reported having had tubal ligation while 15% reported that their husbands had had a vasectomy. *[Chandra, 1998]* Approximately half of female sterilizations in the USA are done in the immediate postpartum period within 48 hours of delivery *[Peterson, 1998]*

EFFECTIVENESS

Failure rates differ by sterilization method and patient's age

Table 32.1 Cumulative 10-year failure rates for voluntary female sterilization methods*

Method	Failure rate (highest rate)	
Post partum salpingectomy	0.8%	For each sterilization method, at ←
Silastic bands	1.8%	least 50% more failures were ascer-
Interval partial salpingectomy	2.0%	tained AFTER 2 YEARS as had been
Bipolar cautery	2.5%	identified in the 2 years immediately
Spring clip	3.7%	following the sterilization procedure

*U.S. Collaborative Review of Sterilization. The risk of pregnancy after tubal sterilization. Am J Obstet Gynecol 1996;174:1161-70.

- Teaching institution rates(above study) may differ from private settings
- Younger women had higher failure rates
- All methods require proper application to maximize effectiveness
- Filshie clip now available (0.9% failure rate - 7 years) *[Chi-Cheng Contraception 1987;* ← *35:171-8]*

MECHANISM

Interruption of fallopian tubes thereby preventing fertilization

LAPAROSCOPIC STERILIZATION

Bipolar cautery:
- Apply to area with no vessels ascending through broad ligament, where the diameter ← of tube similar on either side of damaged area (at least 2 cm from uterotubal junction). Thoroughly cauterize tissue using bipolar cutting current of 25 Watts. Use of an ammeter can confirm tubal destruction. This method has the highest risk of subsequent fistulization and ectopic pregnancy.

Silastic band: (Falope ring, Yoon band)
- Apply over knuckle of tube at least 3 cm from utero-tubal junction. Loop of tube should clearly contain two complete ligaments of tube.

Hulka-Clemens clip (spring clip):
- Spring-loaded clip. Apply to isthmic portion of tube. 1-2 cm distal to cornu at an angle of 90% relative to long axis of tube. High potential for reversibility. Highest failure rate

Filshie clip:
- Hinged titanium with cured silicone rubber clip. Apply to isthmic portion of tube, 1 to 2 cm from cornu. High potential for reversibility

Figure 32.1 Laparoscopic Technique Diagrams

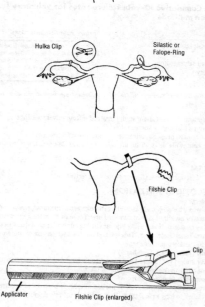

Bipolar Cauterization

in two or three adjacent areas (failure rates are lowest with a triple burn)

Hulka Clip

Silastic or Falope-Ring

Filshie Clip

Clip

Applicator

Filshie Clip (enlarged)

POSTPARTUM OR INTERVAL MINI-LAPAROTOMY METHODS

Pomeroy:
- Ligation at the base of a loop of isthmic portion of tube with plain catgut suture followed by excision of the knuckle of tube

Parkland:
- Excision of segment of isthmic portion of tube after separate ligation of cut ends

Irving:
- Doubly ligate and sever tube. Bury proximal stump into uterus/distal stump into mesosalpinx

Uchida:
- Inject mesenteric part of tube with saline. Divide muscular part of tube/excise 3-5 cm. Bury proximal tube and exteriorize or excise distal tube

Figure 32.2 Postpartum Techniques

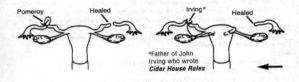

Pomeroy   Healed   Irving*   Healed

*Father of John Irving who wrote *Cider House Rules*

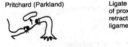

Pritchard (Parkland)

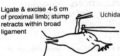

Ligate & excise 4-5 cm of proximal limb; stump retracts within broad ligament   Uchida

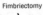

Fimbriectomy

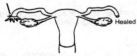

Healed

COST in 1995

Managed-Care Setting	Public Provider Setting
$2500	$1200

ADVANTAGES

Menstrual: None

Sexual/psychological:
- Enhanced enjoyment of sex by reducing worry of pregnancy

Cancers, tumors, and masses:
- Decreased risk of ovarian cancer

Other:
- Permanent
- Highly effective

DISADVANTAGES

Menstrual:
- Data from 9514 women who underwent tubal sterilization by 6 techniques and ← followed for up to 5 years suggest no "post-tubal ligation syndrome" and no increases in the amount or duration of menstrual bleeding or menstrual pain. *[Peterson, 2000]*

Sexual/psychological: Regret may occur
- Some women resist tubal sterilization just as some men resist vasectomy

Cancers, tumors, and masses: None

Other:
- Requires outpatient surgery (most commonly with general anesthesia)
- Expensive in short term
- If failure occurs, higher risk of ectopic pregnancy (10%-65%)
- Does not prevent spread of HIV and STIs
- Not readily reversible

COMPLICATIONS *[Peterson, 1997]*

	Minilaparotomy	Laparoscopy
Minor	11.6%	6.0%
Major	1.5%	0.9%

- Minor complications include infection, wound separation
- Major complications include conversion to laparotomy, hemorrhage, viscus injury
- Major vessel injury risk w/ laparoscopy 3-9/10,000 procedures
- Mortality: 1-2/100,000 procedures (leading cause is general anesthesia)

LONG-TERM RISKS

- Statistically higher risk for subsequent hysterectomy, but only in women who had gynecologic complaints prior to sterilization
- Regret (0.9% - 26.0%) Risk factors include: young age, change in marital status, poverty, minority status, misinformation about permanence; decision made in a hurry

CANDIDATES FOR USE

- Woman who is certain she wants no more children
- Woman over age 21 (only required for Medicaid reimbursement, not for medical requirements)
- Woman with a medical condition that makes pregnancy dangerous
- Woman for whom surgery is considered safe

Adolescents: Not a preferred method, generally higher regret and higher failure rates

PRESTERILIZATION COUNSELING CHECKLIST*

__Discuss vasectomy as an alternative

__Insure patient commitment to having no future children, even if something happened to her current family

__Discuss alternative reversible methods and quote their effectiveness (see algorithm). (IUDs, DMPA, Lunelle, and implants are more effective then some forms of tubal sterilization).

__Describe details of surgery (informed consent later) and possible intraoperative and long-term complications (risk for ectopic pregnancy)

__Stress that procedure must be considered irreversible and that about 10% of women regret their decision.

__Answer all of her questions

__Obtain informed consent - No requirement that spouse must be involved

*Adapted from ACOG Technical Bulletin, April 1996.

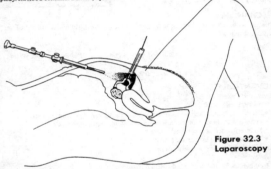

**Figure 32.3
Laparoscopy**

INITIATING METHOD

• Obtain informed consent. Preferable to involve partner in process, but not necessary
• Any time in cycle with certainty of no pregnancy, otherwise follicular timing preferred

FOLLOW-UP

• Follow up in two weeks for post op wound check. Routine annual gynecology exams

MANAGEMENT OF PROBLEMS

• Anesthesia complications, wound infections, intraperitoneal adhesion formation, hydrosalpinx – managed with standard tools

FERTILITY AFTER USE

• Women must desire to be permanently sterile because reversal is costly and failure rates are high. In vitro fertilization may be preferable, but many couples cannot afford this procedure

CHAPTER 33

Male Sterilization: Vasectomy

www.avsc.org or www.plannedparenthood.org

DESCRIPTION

Permanent male contraception. Outpatient surgical procedure. Involves cutting and ligating or cauterizing vas. No-scalpel technique punctures scrotum, delivers vas; ligates or cauterizes vas

EFFECTIVENESS (See Table 13.2, p. 36)

Perfect use failure rate in first year: 0.10%
Typical use failure rate in first year: 0.15%
[Trussell J, Contraceptive Technology, 1998]

> Although vasectomy is safer and potentially more effective than tubal sterilization, as of mid-2000, there are only 4 nations in the world where vasectomies exceed tubal sterilizations: Great Britain, the Netherlands, New Zealand and Bhutan.

MECHANISM

Interrupts vas deferens. Prevents passage of sperm into seminal fluid and into the female reproductive tract

COST

	Managed-Care Setting	Public Provider Setting
	$755.70	$353.28
	[Trussell, 1995; Smith, 1993]	

ADVANTAGES

Menstrual: None
Sexual/psychological:
- Sexual intercourse may be more enjoyable because fear of pregnancy decreased
- Permits man opportunity to take on an important contraceptive role
- No interference during sexual intercourse
- No contraceptive burden for female

Cancers, tumors, and masses: None
Other:
- Simpler, safer and more effective than female sterilization
- Cost-effective
- Convenient
- Shares contraception responsibility with male partner
- No supplies or further clinic visits needed after sperm count has been documented to be zero

DISADVANTAGES

Menstrual: None
Sexual/psychological:
- Some men resist vasectomy fearing that it will interfere with sexual function and because they feel contraception is the woman's responsibility
- Regret at a later time possible
- Will need back-up method until sperm count reaches zero. Female partner may still need contraception if she has other partners or if STI protection needed

Cancers, tumors, and masses: None
Other:
- Does not reduce risk for STIs; will still need to use condom if at risk
- Short-term post-operative discomfort, bruising, and swelling.

- Requires surgical procedure by trained provider

COMPLICATIONS
- Surgically related complaints such as hematoma, bruising, wound infection, or adverse reaction to local anesthesia
- Later regret possible

CANDIDATES FOR USE
Male who: Desires a permanent, effective method of contraception
Adolescents: Not a preferred method

INITIATING METHOD
- Take preoperative history; make general health assessment
- Obtain informed consent. In general, try to involve partner
- Carefully counsel, especially about permanence of method
- Advise patient to bathe genital area and upper thighs prior to surgery; wear clean, loose-fitting clothes to facility; take no medication 24 hours before procedure

PRESCRIBING PRECAUTIONS
- Current infection of penis, prostate, or scrotum
- Current skin infection over incision site
- Fear of needles or scalpels (scalpels not required if no-scalpel vasectomy)

Figure 33.1 Vasectomy

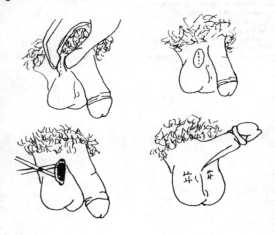

INSTRUCTIONS FOR PATIENT

- Apply ice pack to incision site to decrease swelling and bruising
- Keep area dry for two days – wear snug underwear and pants to provide support where needed
- If any symptoms or signs of infection develop, seek help immediately.
- Return as directed for sperm counts. Use other forms of contraception until sperm count reaches zero

FOLLOW-UP

__Have you had your semen tested for the presence of sperm? If yes, were sperm absent?

PROBLEM MANAGEMENT

Wound infection: Treat with antibiotics. Drain and treat any abscesses

Hematoma: Apply warm moist packs to scrotum. Provide scrotal support

Granuloma: Observe; usually it will resolve itself

Pain at site: If no infection, provide scrotal support and analgesics

Excessive swelling: If large and painful, may require surgery. Provide scrotal support if hematoma

FERTILITY AFTER USE

- Man and woman must both accept that vasectomy is irreversible and permanent
- Microsurgical techniques of reversal now result in pregnancy rates of 50% or above, and in return of sperm to ejaculate in over 90% of men
- Important factors for reversal are
  - skill of microsurgeon
  - length of time from vasectomy
  - presence of antisperm antibodies
  - partner's fertility
  - manner in which vasectomy was performed (amount of vas removed or cauterized)

CHAPTER 34

Future Methods

www.popcouncil.org or www.conrad.org OR
www.plannedparenthood.org/ARTICLES/bcfuture-w.html ←

NEW HORMONAL FORMULATIONS FOR ORAL USE

Several lower-dose COCs are currently available in Europe with EE levels of 10-15 µg and newer progestins that are not derived from androgens but from spironolactone. These new progestins have anti-mineralocorticoid activity and anti-androgenic activity. ←
The first of these new progestins in the U.S. will be drospirinone

Table 34.1 PROGESTIN-ONLY IMPLANTS

NAME	# CAPSULES	HORMONE	LENGTH OF USE	BIODEGRADABLE
Norplant 2	2	Levonorgestrel	5 yrs.	no
Uniplant	1	nomegestrol		
Nestorone	1	nestorone	2 yrs.	
Annuelle	pellets	norethindrone		

VAGINAL DELIVERY SYSTEMS

- NuvaRing: a 5.4 cm diameter flexible ring 4 mm in thickness made from a soft material called EVA (ethylene vinylacetate). NuvaRing releases both EE and the progestin etonogestrel (3-ketodesogestrel) from its core. One ring is placed in vagina for 3 weeks and then removed. The woman uses nothing for 1 week to allow for menstruation. Another ring is placed at the end of the 4 week cycle. Efficacy is generally comparable to COCs; one year failure rate of 0.6% in European study and 1.8% in U.S. study. Steady release and reliable use allows lower circulating levels of hormone than oral route and leads to very regular menses. No pressure problems on vaginal mucosa. Average woman loses very small amount of weight
- Progestin-only vaginal rings: may be worn continuously
- Progesterone daily suppositories

TRANSDERMAL PATCH

- Estrogen/progestin patches (EE and 17-deacetylnorgestimate): Clinical trials completed in US with one version, Ortho-Evra patches (20 cm²) containing ethinyl estradiol and norelgestromin (the primary active metabolite of norgestimate); women use one patch each week for 3 weeks (usually on abdomen or buttocks), then forgo use for one week to allow for menses. Efficacy and side effects similar to OCs. Compliance and ovulation suppression better than with COCs

INTRAUTERINE DEVICES

- Gynefix Copper IUD (Multiload Copper IUD): 6 sleeves of copper on a string that has one end embedded in fundus and other end protruding through cervix for monthly monitoring. IUD has low expulsion rate and cumulative 3-year failure rate of 0.5%

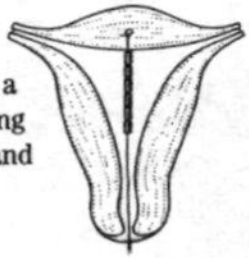

FEMALE BARRIERS

- New prototypes of female condoms
- Lea's shield: silicone rubber diaphragm; one size fits all
- Femcap: silicone rubber cervical cap; 3 sizes
- Protectaid: new vaginal sponges
- Microbicides which are also spermicidal—may not be available for a decade

Figure 34.1
Gynefix intrauterine
copper implant

MALE METHODS

- Male hormonal methods under development often use exogenous progestin or gonadotropin-releasing hormone (GnRH) antagonist to suppress FSH and LH, thereby decreasing spermatogenesis. Replacement testosterone provided
  injectables: progestin + testosterone / GnRH + testosterone
  implants: 2 implant system with GnRH + androgen
- Testosterone (injectable or patch) combined with slow release progestin implant
- Immunocontraception: Methods based on interference of the reproductive process by products of an immune reaction
- "Temporary sterilization"— injecting the vas deferens with a polymer to block sperm
- Anti-sperm compounds, e.g., gossypol from cottonseed oil and Triptolide

NEW EC METHODS: A variety will arise in the future

VACCINES: In phase 1 trials

QUINACRINE STERILIZATION: extremely controversial

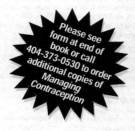

Please see form at end of book or call 404-373-0530 to order additional copies of Managing Contraception

CHAPTER 35

Sexually Transmissible Infections (STIs)
1998 CDC Guidelines for Treatment

Complete guidelines at www.cdc.gov/nchstp/od/nchstp.html

Since women and men seeking contraceptives are also at risk for STIs, we have included in this book information on the treatment of many of the most important STIs. New therapies may be available but are not yet incorporated by CDC into its guidelines. The 2001 CDC Treatment Guidelines are due to be published in the fall of 2001. They will be included in the next edition of *Managing Contraception* (out in June, 2002). Contents:

CLINICAL PREVENTION GUIDELINES

- This section is a summary of selected paragraphs and treatments from the *1998 Guidelines for Sexually Transmitted Diseases* published by the CDC *[CDC, 1998]*
- The specific recommendations presented here are from that document
- Both partners should get tested for STIs, including HIV, before initiating sexual intercourse
- A new condom should be used for each act of intercourse

Prevention Methods
- *Male Condoms*
  - Used consistently and correctly, condoms are effective in preventing many STIs, including HIV
  - Failure usually results from inconsistent or incorrect use, rather than condom breakage

- *Female Condoms*
  - Laboratory studies indicate that the female condom (Reality) is an effective mechanical barrier to viruses, including HIV
  - Used consistently and correctly, the female condom should substantially reduce risk for STIs

- *Condoms and Spermicides*
  - Whether condoms used with vaginal application of spermicide are more effective than condoms used without vaginal spermicides has not been determined
  - Therefore, the consistent use of condoms, with or without spermicidal lubricant or vaginal application of spermicide, is recommended

- However, vaginal spermicides offer no protection against HIV infection, and spermicides are not recommended for HIV prevention
- Diaphragm use has been demonstrated to provide some protection against cervical gonorrhea, chlamydia, and trichomoniasis
- Vaginal sponges or diaphragms should not be assumed to protect women against HIV infection

- **Nonbarrier Contraception, Surgical Sterilization, and Hysterectomy**
  - Hormonal contraception (e.g., oral contraceptives, Norplant, and Depo-Provera) has been associated in some cohort studies with cervical STIs and increased acquisition of HIV; however, data concerning this finding are inconsistent
  - Women who use hormonal or intrauterine contraception, have been surgically sterilized, or have had hysterectomies should still be counseled on the use of condoms for STI protection

SPECIAL POPULATIONS

Pregnant Women

- **Recommended Screening Tests**
  - Syphilis: all pregnant women at first prenatal visit
  - Hepatitis B surface antigen (HbsAg): all pregnant women first visit
  - *Neisseria gonorrhoeae:* first visit for women at risk or living in an area of high prevalence
  - *Chlamydia trachomatis:* third trimester for women at increased risk (i.e., women aged <25 years and women who have a new or more than one sex partner or whose partner has other partners)
  - HIV screening test: offered to all pregnant women at the first prenatal visit
  - Bacterial vaginosis (BV): early second trimester for asymptomatic patients at high risk for preterm labor. Current evidence does not support universal testing for BV
  - Papanicolaou (Pap) smear: first visit if no Pap smear has been documented during the preceding year

- **Other Concerns (Other STI-related Concerns are to Be Considered as Follow:)**
  - Pregnant women who have either primary genital herpes infection, HBV, primary cytomegalovirus (CMV) infection, or Group B streptococcal infection and women who have syphilis and who are allergic to penicillin may need to be referred to an expert for management
  - HbsAg-positive pregnant women should be reported to the local and/or state health department; household and sexual contacts of HbsAg-positive women should be tested and immunized if negative
  - In the absence of lesions during the third trimester, routine serial culture for herpes simplex virus (HSV) is not indicated for women who have a history of recurrent genital herpes. However, obtaining cultures from such women at the time of delivery may be useful in guiding neonatal management. Prophylactic cesarean section is not indicated for women who do not have active genital lesions at the time of delivery
  - The presence of genital warts is not an indication for cesarean section unless size obstructs delivery in labor (rare)

Adolescents

- With limited exceptions, all U.S. adolescents can consent to the confidential diagnosis and treatment of STIs. See Table 6.1, p. 16
- Medical care for STIs can be provided to adolescents without parental consent or knowledge
- Providers should appreciate how important confidentiality is to adolescents

DISEASES CHARACTERIZED BY GENITAL ULCERS

Management of Patients Who Have Genital Ulcers

- In the United States, most young, sexually active patients who have genital ulcers have genital herpes, syphilis, or chancroid. Each disease has been associated with an increased risk for HIV infection
- The evaluation of all patients who have genital ulcers should include a serologic test for syphilis and diagnostic evaluation for herpes. Specific tests (to be used with clinical assessment) for the evaluation of genital ulcers include the following:
  - Dark-field examination or direct immunofluorescence test for *Treponema pallidum*
  - Culture or antigen test for HSV
  - Culture for *Haemophilus ducreyi*
- HIV testing should be a) performed in the management of patients who have genital ulcers caused by *T. pallidum* or *H. ducreyi* and b) considered for those who have ulcers caused by HSV

CHANCROID (SHAN–kroyd)

Organism: H. ducreyi.

Diagnosis: Culture on special medium of *H. ducreyi*, or if the following criteria are met: a) patient has 1 or more ulcers; b) no evidence of syphilis on lab exam after at least 7 days; c) the clinical picture is typical of chancroid and d) test for HSV is negative.

Treatment: Recommended Regimens

Azithromycin	1 g orally in a single dose, OR
Ceftriaxone	250 mg intramuscularly (IM) in a single dose, OR
Ciprofloxacin	500 mg orally twice a day for 3 days, OR
Erythromycin base	500 mg orally four times a day for 7 days.

Follow-up: Re-examine in 3-7 days. If no improvement consider whether a) the diagnosis is correct, b) the patient is coinfected with another STI, c)the patient is infected with HIV, d) the treatment was not taken as instructed, or e) the *H. ducreyi* strain causing the infection is resistant to the prescribed antimicrobial.

- *The time required for complete healing:*
  - Depends on the size of the ulcer; large ulcers may require >2 weeks
  - Healing is slower for some uncircumcised men who have ulcers under the foreskin
  - Resolution of fluctuant lymphadenopathy is slower than that of ulcers and may require drainage, even during otherwise successful therapy
  - Although needle aspiration of buboes is a simple procedure, incision and drainage of buboes may be preferred because of less need for subsequent drainage procedures

Management of Sex Partners: Should be examined and treated regardless of symptoms if they had sexual contact within 10 days of the onset of symptoms.

Special Considerations: Pregnancy. The safety of azithromycin for pregnant and lactating women has not been established. Ciprofloxacin is contraindicated during pregnancy. No adverse effects of chancroid on pregnancy outcome or on the fetus have been reported.

GENITAL HERPES SIMPLEX VIRAL (HSV) INFECTION (Her–pes)

Most persons shed the virus intermittently and are unaware that they are infected and are asymptomatic at the time of transmission.

Organisms: HSV-1 and HSV-2.

Diagnosis: See complete *1998 CDC Guidelines* or *Contraceptive Technology*

Counseling: Counseling of these patients should include the following:
- Patients should be advised to abstain from sexual activity when lesions or prodromal symptoms are present and encouraged to inform their sex partners that they have genital herpes
- Use condoms during all sexual exposures with new or uninfected sex partners
- Sexual transmission of HSV can occur during asymptomatic periods
- The risk for neonatal infection should be explained to all patients, including men. Childbearing-aged women who have genital herpes should be advised to inform health-care providers who care for them during pregnancy about the HSV infection
- Patients having a first episode of genital herpes should be advised that a) episodic antiviral therapy during recurrent episodes might shorten the duration of lesions and b) suppressive antiviral therapy can ameliorate or prevent recurrent outbreaks

Treatment: 5% to 30% of first-episode cases of genital herpes are caused by HSV-1, but clinical recurrences are much less frequent for HSV-1 than HSV-2 genital infection.

• HSV, Recommended Regimens for First Clinical Infection

Acyclovir	400 mg orally three times a day for 7-10 days, OR
Acyclovir	200 mg orally five times a day for 7-10 days, OR
Famciclovir	250 mg orally three times a day for 7-10 days, OR
Valacyclovir	1 g orally twice a day for 7-10 days.

• HSV, Recommended Regimens for Episodic Recurrent Infection

Acyclovir	400 mg orally three times a day for 5 days, OR
Acyclovir	200 mg orally five times a day for 5 days, OR
Acyclovir	800 mg orally twice a day for 5 days, OR
Famciclovir	125 mg orally twice a day for 5 days, OR
Valacyclovir	500 mg orally twice a day for 5 days.

• HSV, Recommended Regimens for Daily Suppressive Therapy

Acyclovir	400 mg orally twice a day, OR
Famciclovir	250 mg orally twice a day, OR
Valacyclovir	250 mg orally twice a day, OR
Valacyclovir	500 mg orally once a day, OR
Valacyclovir	1000 mg orally once a day.

- Valacyclovir 500 mg once a day appears less effective than other valacyclovir dosing regimens in patients who have very frequent recurrences (i.e., >10 episodes per year)
- Valacyclovir and famciclovir appear to be comparable to acyclovir in clinical outcome
- However, valacyclovir and famciclovir may provide increased ease in administration

Severe Disease: IV therapy should be provided for patients who have severe disease or complications necessitating hospitalization, such as disseminated infection, pneumonitis, hepatitis, or complications of the central nervous system (e.g., meningitis or encephalitis).

• HSV, Recommended Regimen for Persons with Severe Disease

Acyclovir	5-10 mg/kg body weight IV every 8 hours for 5-7 days until clinical resolution is attained.

Special Considerations:
- *Pregnancy*
  - The safety of systemic acyclovir and valacyclovir therapy in pregnant women has not been established
  - Women who receive acyclovir or valacyclovir during pregnancy should be reported to the CDC registry; telephone **1-800-331-3435**

- Current registry findings do not indicate an increased risk for major birth defects after acyclovir treatment
- Prenatal exposure to valacyclovir and famciclovir is too limited to provide useful information on pregnancy outcomes
- *Perinatal Infection*
  - The risk for transmission to the neonate from an infected mother is high (30% - 50%) among women who acquire genital herpes near the time of delivery and is low (3%) among women who have a history of recurrent herpes at term and women who acquire genital HSV during the first half of pregnancy
  - Therefore, prevention of neonatal herpes should emphasize prevention of acquisition of genital HSV infection during late pregnancy
  - Susceptible women whose partners have oral or genital HSV infection, or those whose sex partners' infection status is unknown, should be counseled to avoid unprotected genital and oral sexual contact during late pregnancy
  - The results of viral cultures during pregnancy do not predict viral shedding at the time of delivery, and such cultures are not indicated routinely
  - At the onset of labor, all women should be examined and carefully questioned about whether they have symptoms of HSV. Infants of women who do not have symptoms or signs of HSV infection or its prodrome may be delivered vaginally
  - Cesarean delivery does not completely eliminate the risk for HSV infection in the neonate

GRANULOMA INGUINALE (DONOVANOSIS) (gran-u-LO-ma in-gwi-NAL-e, don-o-van-O-sis)

Organism: *Calymmatobacterium granulomatis* is an intracellular, gram-negative bacterium. It is seen rarely in the USA. Presents as a painless, progressive, vascular, ulcerative lesion with regional lymphadenopathy.

Diagnosis: Visualization of Donovan bodies from tissue of lesion

Treatment: Appears to halt progressive destruction of tissue. Prolonged duration of therapy often required to enable granulation and re-epithelialization of the ulcers. Therapy should be continued until all lesions have healed completely.

- *Granuloma Inguinale, Recommended Regimens*

Trimethoprim-
sulfamethoxazole....................One double-strength tablet orally twice a day for a minimum of 3 weeks, OR

Doxycycline.............................100 mg orally twice a day for a minimum or 3 weeks.

- *Granuloma Inguinale, Alternative Regimens*

Ciprofloxacin..........................750 mg orally twice a day for a minimum of 3 weeks, OR

Erythromycin base.................500 mg orally four times a day for a minimum of 3 weeks (for use during pregnancy).

- For any of the above regimens, the addition of an aminoglycoside (gentamicin 1 mg/kg IV every 8 hours) should be considered if lesions do not respond within the first few days of therapy

LYMPHOGRANULOMA VENEREUM (LGV) (lim-fo-gran-u-LO-ma ve-nar-E-um)

This is a rare disease in the USA, most frequently manifested in heterosexual men as unilateral tender inguinal nodes and in women and homosexual men with proctocolitis, or inflammatory involvement or perirectal or perianal fistulas or strictures

Organism: Invasive strains L1, L2, or L3 of *Chlamydia trachomatis.*
Diagnosis: Serological and exclusion of other ulcerative lesions or those with lymphadenopathy.
Treatment: Treatment cures infection and prevents ongoing tissue damage, although tissue reaction can result in scarring. Buboes may require aspiration through intact skin or incision and drainage to prevent the formation of inguinal/femoral ulcerations.

• *LGV, Recommended Regimen*
Doxycycline............................. 100 mg orally twice a day for 21 days OR
Erythromycin base..................500 mg orally four times a day for 21 days

SYPHILIS   (SIF-i-lis)

Organism: *Treponema pallidum* (tre-po-NE-ma PAL-e-dum)
Diagnosis:
- See most recent CDC Guidelines or ***Contraceptive Technology***

Treatment:
- Parenteral penicillin G is preferred drug for treatment of all stages of syphilis. The preparation(s) used (i.e., benzathine, aqueous procaine, or aqueous crystalline), the dosage, and the length of treatment depend on the stage and clinical manifestations of disease
- Parenteral penicillin G is the only therapy with documented efficacy for neurosyphilis or for syphilis during pregnancy. Patients who report a penicillin allergy, including pregnant women with syphilis in any stage and patients with neurosyphilis, should be desensitized and treated with penicillin
- The Jarisch-Herxheimer reaction is an acute febrile reaction often accompanied by headache, myalgia, and other symptoms that might occur within the first 24 hours after any therapy for syphilis; patients should be advised of this possible adverse reaction

PRIMARY AND SECONDARY SYPHILIS:

• *Recommended Regimen for Adults*
Benzathine penicillin G....... 2.4 million units IM in a single dose

Other Management Considerations: All patients who have syphilis should be tested for HIV infection. In geographic areas in which the prevalence of HIV is high, patients who have primary syphilis should be retested for HIV after 3 months if the first HIV test result was negative.
Follow-up: Serologic test titers may decline more slowly for patients who previously had syphilis. Patients should be reexamined clinically and serologically at both 6 months and 12 months; also see complete *1998 CDC Guidelines* for more detail.
Management of Sex Partners: *Sexual transmission of* T. pallidum *occurs only when mucocutaneous syphilitic lesions are present;* such manifestations are uncommon after the first year of infection. However, persons exposed sexually to a patient who has syphilis in any stage should be evaluated clinically and serologically according to CDC.
Special Considerations
- *Penicillin Allergy:* Nonpregnant penicillin-allergic patients who have primary or secondary syphilis should be treated with one of the following regimens. Close follow-up of such patients is essential.

• *Recommended Regimens*
Doxycycline...............................100 mg orally twice a day for 2 weeks, OR
Tetracycline.............................500 mg orally four times a day for 2 weeks.

- Pregnant patients who are allergic to penicillin should be desensitized, if necessary, and treated with penicillin.

LATENT SYPHILIS:
See most recent CDC Guidelines or *Contraceptive Technology*

TERTIARY SYPHILIS:
See most recent CDC Guidelines or *Contraceptive Technology*

DISEASES CHARACTERIZED BY URETHRITIS AND CERVICITIS

Management of Patients Who Have Nongonococcal Urethritis
Diagnosis: Testing for chlamydia is strongly recommended because of the increased utility and availability of highly sensitive and specific testing methods and because a specific diagnosis might improve compliance and partner notification.
Treatment:

- *Nongonococcal Urethritis, Recommended Regimens*
Azithromycin...........................1 g orally in a single dose, OR
Doxycycline............................100 mg orally twice a day for 7 days.

- *Nongonococcal Urethritis, Alternative Regimens*
Erythromycin base.................500 mg orally four times a day for 7 days, OR
Erythromycin ethylsuccinate.....800 mg orally four times a day for 7 days, OR
Ofloxacin................................300 mg twice a day for 7 days.

Follow-up: If symptoms persist, patients should be instructed to return for reevaluation and to abstain from sexual intercourse even if they have completed the prescribed therapy.
Partner Referral: Patients should refer all sex partners within the preceding 60 days for evaluation and treatment.

- *Recurrent/Persistent Urethritis, Recommended Treatment*
Metronidazole..........................2 g orally in a single dose, PLUS
Erythromycin base.................500 mg orally four times a day for 7 days, OR
Erythromycin ethylsuccinate....800 mg orally four times a day for 7 days.

CHLAMYDIAL INFECTION IN ADOLESCENTS AND ADULTS

Several important sequelae can result from *Chlamydia trachomatis* (kla-MID-e-a tra-KO-ma-tis) infection in women; the most serious of these include PID, ectopic pregnancy, and infertility. Some women who have apparently uncomplicated cervical infection already have subclinical upper reproductive tract infection.
Diagnosis: See complete *1998 CDC Guidelines* or *Contraceptive Technology*
Treatment:

- Treatment of infected patients prevents transmission to sex partners and, for infected pregnant women, might prevent transmission to infants during birth
- Treatment of sex partners helps to prevent reinfection of the index patient and infection of other partners
- Coinfection with *C. trachomatis* often occurs among patients who have gonococcal infection; therefore, presumptive treatment of such patients for chlamydia is appropriate (see GONOCOCCAL INFECTION, Dual Therapy for Gonococcal and Chlamydial Infection, p 149)
- The following recommended treatment regimens and the alternative regimens cure infection and usually relieve symptoms:

- *Chlamydia Infection, Recommended Regimens*
  Azithromycin............................1 g orally in a single dose, OR
  Doxycycline..............................100 mg orally twice a day for 7 days.

- *Chlamydia Infection, Alternative Regimens*
  Erythromycin base..................500 mg orally four times a day for 7 days, OR
  Erythromycin ethylsuccinate......800 mg orally four times a day for 7 days, OR
  Ofloxacin.................................300 mg orally twice a day for 7 days.

Follow-up: Patients do not need to be retested for chlamydia after completing treatment with doxycycline or azithromycin unless symptoms persist or reinfection is suspected because these therapies are highly efficacious.

Management of Sex Partners: Patients should be instructed to refer their sex partners for evaluation, testing, and treatment, if they had sexual contact with the patient during the 60 days preceding onset of symptoms in the patient or diagnosis of chlamydia.

Special Considerations:

- *Pregnancy:*
  - Doxycycline and ofloxacin are contraindicated for pregnant women
  - The safety and efficacy of azithromycin use in pregnant and lactating women have not been established
  - Repeat testing, preferably by culture, 3 weeks after completion of therapy with the following regimens is recommended because a) none of these regimens is highly efficacious and b) frequent side effects of erythromycin may discourage patient compliance

- *Recommended Regimens for Pregnant Women*
  Erythromycin base..................500 mg orally four times a day for 7 days. OR
  Amoxicillin............................500 mg orally three times a day for 7 days.

- *Alternative Regimens for Pregnant Women*
  Erythromycin base..................250 mg orally four times a day for 14 days. OR
  Erythromycin ethylsuccinate.....800 mg orally four times a day for 7 days, OR
  Erythromycin ethylsuccinate.....400 mg orally four times a day for 14 days, OR
  Azithromycin............................1 g orally in a single dose.

- Note: Erythromycin estolate is contraindicated during pregnancy because of drug-related hepatotoxicity. Preliminary data indicate that azithromycin may be safe and effective.

GONOCOCCAL INFECTION

DUAL THERAPY FOR GONOCOCCAL AND CHLAMYDIAL INFECTIONS

Patients infected with *N. gonorrhoeae* often are coinfected with *C. trachomatis*; this finding led to the recommendation that patients treated for gonococcal infection also be treated routinely with a regimen effective against uncomplicated genital *C. trachomatis* infection.

Uncomplicated Gonococcal Infections of the Cervix, Urethra, and Rectum

- *Recommended Regimens*
  Cefixime....................................400 mg orally in a single dose OR
  Ceftriaxone..............................125 mg IM in a single dose, OR
  Ciprofloxacin...........................500 mg orally in a single dose, OR
  Ofloxacin.................................400 mg orally in a single dose, OR
  Azithromycin............................1 g orally in a single dose, OR
  Doxycycline..............................100 mg orally twice a day for 7 days.

Uncomplicated Gonococcal Infections of the Cervix, Urethra, and Rectum
- **Alternative Regimens**

Spectinomycin........................2 g IM in a single dose. Spectinomycin is effective, but it is expensive and must be injected. It is useful for treatment of patients who cannot tolerate cephalosporins and quinolones.

Single-dose cephalosporin....regimens other than cefritaxone 125 mg IM and cefixime 400 mg include a) ceftizoxime 500 mg IM, b) cefotaxime 500 mg IM, c) cefotetan 1g IM, and d) cefoxitin 2 g IM with probenicid 1 g orally.

Single-dose quinolone............regimens include enoxacin 400 mg orally, lomefloxacin 400 mg orally, and norfloxacin 800 mg orally. None of the regimens appears to offer any advantage over ciprofloxacin or ofloxacin.

- Many other antimicrobials are active against *N. gonorrhoeae*
- Azithromycin 2 g orally is effective against uncomplicated gonococcal infection, but it is expensive and causes gastrointestinal distress too often to be recommended for treatment of gonorrhea
- An oral dose of 1 g azithromycin is insufficiently effective (93%)

Uncomplicated Gonococcal Infection of the Pharynx
- Gonococcal infections of the pharynx are more difficult to eradicate than infections at urogenital and anorectal sites
- Few antigonococcal regimens can reliably cure such infections >90% of the time
- Although chlamydial coinfection of the pharynx is unusual, coinfection at genital sites sometimes occurs. Therefore, treatment for both gonorrhea and chlamydia is suggested

- **Recommended Regimen**

Ceftriaxone...............................125 mg IM in a single dose, OR

Ciprofloxacin...........................500 mg orally in a single dose, OR

Ofloxacin...................................400 mg orally in a single dose, OR

Azithromycin............................1 g orally in a single dose, OR

Doxycycline...............................100 mg orally twice a day for 7 days.

Management of Sex Partners: All sex partners of patients who have *N. gonorrhea* infection should be evaluated and treated for *N. gonorrhea* and *C. trachomatis* infections if their last sexual contact with the patient was within 60 days before onset of symptoms or diagnosis

Special Considerations:
- Pregnant women should not be treated with quinolones or tetracyclines
- Pregnant women infected with *N. gonorrhoeae* should be treated with a recommended or alternate cephalosporin
- Women who cannot tolerate a cephalosporin should be administered a single 2-g dose of spectinomycin IM
- Either erythromycin or amoxicillin is recommended for treatment of presumptive or diagnosed *C. trachomatis* infection during pregnancy (see CHLAMYDIAL INFECTION, p. 145)

DISEASES CHARACTERIZED BY VAGINAL DISCHARGE

Management of Patients Who Have Vaginal Infections

- Vaginitis is usually characterized by a vaginal discharge or vulvar itching and irritation; a vaginal odor may be present
- The three diseases most frequently associated with vaginal discharge are trichomoniasis (caused by *T. vaginalis*), BV (caused by a replacement of the normal vaginal flora by an overgrowth of anaerobic microorganisms and *Gardnerella vaginalis*), and candidiasis (usually caused by *Candida albicans*)
- Mucopurulent cervicitis caused by *C. trachomatis* or *N. gonorrhoeae* can sometimes cause vaginal discharge
- Vaginitis is diagnosed by pH and microscopic examination of fresh samples of the discharge
- The pH of the vaginal secretions can be determined by narrow-range pH paper for the elevated pH typical of BV or trichomoniasis (i.e., pH of >4.5)
- One way to examine the discharge is to dilute a sample in one to two drops of 0.9% normal saline solution on one slide and 10% potassium hydroxide (KOH) solution on a second slide. Always prepare saline slide first.
- An amine odor detected immediately after applying KOH suggests BV
- A cover slip is placed on each slide, which is then examined under a microscope at low and high-dry power. The motile *T. vaginalis* or the clue cells of BV usually are identified easily in the saline specimen
- The yeast or pseudohyphae of *Candida* species are more easily identified in the KOH specimen
- The presence of objective signs of vulvar inflammation in the absence of vaginal pathogens, along with a minimal amount of discharge, suggests the possibility of mechanical, chemical, allergic, or other noninfectious irritation of the vulva
- Culture for *T. vaginalis* is more sensitive than microscopic examination
- Laboratory testing fails to identify the cause of vaginitis among a substantial minority of women

BACTERIAL VAGINOSIS (BV)

- BV is a clinical syndrome resulting from replacement of the normal H_2O_2 producing *Lactobacillus* sp. in the vagina with high concentrations of anaerobic bacteria (e.g., *Prevotella* sp. and *Mobiluncus* sp.), *G. vaginalis*, and *Mycoplasma hominis*
- BV is the most prevalent cause of vaginal discharge or malodor
- Half of women whose illnesses meet the clinical criteria for BV are asymptomatic. It is not necessarily an STI
- Treatment of male sex partner has not been beneficial in preventing recurrence

Diagnostic Considerations: BV can be diagnosed by the use of clinical criteria meeting three of the following symptoms or signs:

   a. A homogeneous, white, noninflammatory discharge that smoothly coats the vaginal walls
   b. The presence of clue cells on microscopic examination
   c. A pH of vaginal fluid >4.5
   d. A fishy odor of vaginal discharge before or after addition of 10% KOH (i.e., the whiff test)

Treatment: The principal goal of therapy is to relieve vaginal symptoms and signs of infection. All women with symptoms require treatment, regardless of pregnancy status

• BV, Recommended Regimens for Nonpregnant Women
Metronidazole..................500 mg orally twice a day for 7 days, OR
Clindamycin cream..............2%, one full applicator (5 g) intravaginally at bedtime for 7 days, OR
Metronidazole gel.............0.75%, one full applicator (5 g) intravaginally, twice a day for 5 days.

- Patients should be advised to avoid consuming alcohol during treatment with metronidazole and for 24 hours thereafter. Clindamycin cream is oil-based and might weaken latex condoms and diaphragms

- **BV, Alternative Regimens**

Metronidazole..........................2 g orally in a single dose, OR

Clindamycin..........................300 mg orally twice a day for 7 days.

- Metronidazole 2 g single-dose therapy is an alternative regimen because of its lower efficacy for BV
- FDA has approved both metronidazole 750-mg extended release tablets once daily for 7 days and metronidazole gel 0.75% once daily intravaginally for 5 days for treatment of BV. However, data concerning clinical equivalency of these regimens with other regimens have not been published. Some health-care providers remain concerned about the possible teratogenicity of metronidazole, which has been suggested by animal experiments; however, a recent meta-analysis does not indicate teratogenicity in humans

Follow-up:
- Follow-up visits are unnecessary if symptoms resolve. Recurrence is not unusual
- Because treatment of BV in high-risk pregnant women who are asymptomatic might prevent adverse pregnancy outcomes, a follow-up evaluation, at 1 month after completion of treatment, should be considered

Management of Sex Partners: Routine treatment of sex partners is not recommended

Special Considerations:

- *Allergy or Intolerance to the Recommended Therapy:*
  - Clindamycin cream is preferred in case of allergy or intolerance to metronidazole Metronidazole gel can be considered for patients who do not tolerate systemic metronidazole, but patients allergic to oral metronidazole should not be administered metronidazole vaginally

- *Pregnancy:*
  - BV has been associated with adverse pregnancy outcomes (i.e., premature rupture of the membranes, preterm labor, and preterm birth)
  - Organisms found in increased concentration in BV also are frequently present in postpartum or post-cesarean endometritis
  - Treatment of BV in high-risk pregnant women (i.e., those who have previously delivered a premature infant) who are asymptomatic might reduce preterm delivery. Screen and treat those with BV at the earliest part of the second trimester
  - The recommended regimen is metronidazole 250 mg orally three times a day for 7 days
  - The alternative regimens are a) metronidazole 2 g orally in a single dose or b) clindamycin 300 mg orally twice a day for 7 days
  - Low-risk pregnant women (i.e., those who previously have not had a premature delivery) who have symptomatic BV should be treated to relieve symptoms. Recommended regimen is metronidazole 250 mg orally three times a day for 7 days
  - Lower doses of medication are recommended for pregnant women to minimize exposure to the fetus. Data are limited concerning the use of metronidazole vaginal gel during pregnancy. Use of clindamycin vaginal cream during pregnancy is not recommended because two randomized trials indicated an increase in the number of preterm deliveries among pregnant women who were treated with this medication

Other: The bacterial flora that characterize BV have been recovered from the endometria and salpinges of women who have PID

TRICHOMONIASIS

Diagnosis:

- Trichomoniasis is caused by the protozoan *T. vaginalis,* easily identified on a wet smear Most men who are infected do not have symptoms of infection, although a minority of men have nongonococcal urethritis
- Many women do have symptoms of infection, characteristically a diffuse, malodorous, yellow-green discharge with vulvar irritation; many women have fewer symptoms
- Vaginal trichomoniasis might be associated with adverse pregnancy outcomes, particularly premature rupture of the membranes and preterm delivery

Treatment:

- ***Trichomoniasis, Recommended Regimen***

  Metronidazole..........................2 g orally in a single dose.

- ***Trichomoniasis, Alternative Regimen***

  Metronidazole..........................500 mg twice a day for 7 days.

- Metronidazole is the only oral medication available in the United States
- In randomized clinical trials, the recommended metronidazole regimens have resulted in cure rates of approximately 90% - 95%; ensuring treatment of sex partners might increase the cure rate. Treatment of patients and sex partners results in relief of microbiologic cure, and reduction of transmission
- Metronidazole gel is approved for treatment of BV, but, like other topically applied antimicrobials that are unlikely to achieve therapeutic levels in the urethra or perivaginal glands, it is considerably less efficacious for treatment than oral preparations of metronidazole and is not recommended

Follow-up:

- Unnecessary for men and women who become asymptomatic after treatment or who are initially asymptomatic
- Infections with strains of *T. vaginalis* that have diminished susceptibility to metronidazole can occur; however, most of these organisms respond to higher doses of metronidazole
- If treatment failure occurs with either regimen, the patient should be retreated with metronidazole 500 mg twice a day for 7 days
- If treatment failure occurs repeatedly, the patient should be treated with a single, 2-g dose of metronidazole once a day for 3-5 days

Special Considerations:

- *Allergy, Intolerance, or Adverse Reactions:* Effective alternatives to therapy with metronidazole are not available. Patients who are allergic to metronidazole can be managed by desensitization
- *Pregnancy:* Patients may be treated with 2 g of metronidazole in a single dose
- *HIV Infection:* Patients who have trichomoniasis and also are infected with HIV should receive the same treatment regimen as those who are HIV negative

VULVOVAGINAL CANDIDIASIS (VVC)

- Vulvovaginal candidiasis (VVC) is caused by *C. albicans* or, occasionally, by other *Candida* sp., *Torulopsis* sp., or other yeasts
- An estimated 75% of women will have at least one episode of VVC
- A small percentage of women (i.e., probably <5%) experience recurrent VVC
- Typical symptoms of VVC include pruritus and vaginal discharge
- Other symptoms may include vaginal soreness, vulvar burning, dyspareunia, and external dysuria
- None of these symptoms is specific for VVC

Diagnostic Considerations:

- A diagnosis of *Candida* vaginitis is suggested clinically by pruritus and erythema in the vulvo-vaginal area; a white discharge may occur, as may vulvar edema
- The diagnosis can be made in a woman who has signs and symptoms of vaginitis, and when either a) a wet preparation or Gram stain of vaginal discharge demonstrates yeasts or pseudohyphae or b) a culture or other test yields a positive result for a yeast species
- *Candida* vaginitis is associated with a normal vaginal pH (<4.5)
- Use of 10% KOH in wet preparations improves the visualization of yeast and mycelia by disrupting cellular material that might obscure the yeast or pseudohyphae
- Identifying *Candida* by culture in the absence of symptoms should not lead to treatment because 10%-20% of women usually harbor *Candida* sp. and other yeasts in the vagina. VVC can occur concomitantly with STIs or frequently following antibacterial vaginal or systemic therapy

Treatment: Topical formulations effectively treat VVC. The topically applied azole drugs are more effective than nystatin. Treatment with azoles results in relief of symptoms and negative cultures among 80%-90% of patients who complete therapy.

- **VVC, Recommended Regimens**
- *Intravaginal agents:*

Butoconazole..........................2% cream 5 g intravaginally for 3 days,* **OR**
Clotrimazole..........................1% cream 5 g intravaginally for 7-14 days,* **OR**
Clotrimazole..........................100-mg vaginal tablet for 7 days,* **OR**
Clotrimazole..........................100-mg vaginal tablet, two tablets for 3 days,* **OR**
Clotrimazole..........................500-mg vaginal tablet, one tablet in a single application,* **OR**
Miconazole..........................2% cream 5 g intravaginally for 7 days,* **OR**
Miconazole..........................200-mg vaginal suppository, one suppository for 3 days,* **OR**
Miconazole..........................100-mg vaginal suppository, one suppository for 7 days,* **OR**
Nystatin..........................100,000-u vaginal tablet, one tablet for 14 days, **OR**
Tioconazole..........................6.5% ointment 5 g intravaginally in a single application,* **OR**
Terconazole..........................0.4% cream 5 g intravaginally for 7 days,* **OR**
Terconazole..........................0.8% cream 5 g intravaginally for 3 days,* **OR**
Terconazole..........................80-mg vaginal suppository, one suppository for 3 days.* **OR**

- *Oral agent:*

Fluconazole..........................150-mg oral tablet, one tablet in single dose.

*These creams and suppositories are oil-based and may weaken latex condoms and diaphragms.

- **VVC, Alternative Regimens**
- Several trials have demonstrated that oral azole agents (ketoconazole and itraconazole) might be as effective as topical agents
- The ease of administering oral agents is an advantage over topical therapies
- However, the potential for toxicity associated with using a systemic drug, particularly ketoconazole, must be considered

Follow-up: Patients should be instructed to return for follow-up visits only if symptoms persist or recur

Management of Sex Partners: None; VVC usually is not acquired through sexual intercourse

Special Considerations:
- *Pregnancy:* VVC often occurs during pregnancy. Only topical azole therapies should be used to treat pregnant women. Of those treatments that have been investigated for use during pregnancy, the most effective are butoconazole, clotrimazole, miconazole, and terconazole. Many experts recommend 7 days of therapy during pregnancy
- *HIV Infection:* Studies are in progress to confirm an alleged increase in incidence of VVC in HIV-infected women

PELVIC INFLAMMATORY DISEASE (PID) (see Table 13.1, page 35)

- PID comprises a spectrum of inflammatory disorders of the upper female genital tract, including any combination of endometritis, salpingitis, tuboovarian abscess, and pelvic peritonitis
- Sexually transmitted organisms, especially *N. gonorrhoeae* and *C. trachomatis*, are implicated in most cases; however, microorganisms that can be part of the vaginal flora (e.g., anaerobes, *G. vaginalis*, *H. influenzae*, enteric gram negative rods, and *Streptococcus agalactiae*) also can cause PID
- In addition, *M. hominis* and *U. urealyticum* may also be etiologic agents

Diagnostic Considerations: See complete *1998 CDC Guidelines (www.cdc.gov).* Empiric treatment should be initiated in sexually active young women and others at risk for STIs if all the following **minimum criteria** are present and no other cause(s) for the illness can be identified:
- Lower abdominal tenderness
- Adnexal tenderness, and
- Cervical motion tenderness

Treatment: Must provide empiric, broad-spectrum coverage of likely pathogens Antimicrobial coverage should include *N. gonorrhea*, *C. trachomatis*, anaerobes, gram-negative facultative bacteria, and streptococci
- *Criteria for HOSPITALIZATION based on observational data and theoretical concerns:*
  - Surgical emergencies such as appendicitis cannot be excluded
  - Patient is pregnant
  - Patient does not respond clinically to oral antimicrobial therapy
  - Patient is unable to follow or tolerate an outpatient oral regimen
  - Patient has severe illness, nausea and vomiting, or high fever
  - Patient has a tuboovarian abscess; or
  - Patient is immunodeficient (i.e., has HIV infection with low CD4 counts, is taking immunosuppressive therapy, or has another disease)

Most clinicians favor at least 24 hours of direct inpatient observation for patients who have tuboovarian abscesses. After that, parenteral therapy should have reduced the risk of abcess progression or rupture

- *PID, Parenteral Regimen A*

Cefotetan	2 g IV every 12 hours, **OR**
Cefoxitin	2 g IV every 6 hours, **PLUS**
Doxycycline	100 mg IV or orally every 12 hours.

- Because of pain associated with infusion, doxycycline should be administered orally when possible, even when the patient is hospitalized
- Both oral and IV administration of doxycycline provide similar bioavailability
- When tuboovarian abscess is present, many health-care providers use clindamycin or metronidazole with doxycycline for continued therapy rather than doxycycline alone, because it provides more effective anaerobic coverage

- **PID, Parenteral Regimen B**

Clindamycin............................ 900 mg IV every 8 hours, **PLUS**

Gentamicin............................loading dose IV or IM (2 mg/kg of body weight) followed by a maintenance dose (1.5 mg/kg) every 8 hours. Single daily dosing may be substituted.)

- Although use of a single daily dose of gentamicin has not been evaluated for the treatment of PID, it is efficacious in analogous situations
- Parenteral therapy may be discontinued 24 hours after a patient improves clinically, and continuing oral therapy should consist of doxycycline 100 mg orally twice a day or clindamycin 450 mg orally four times a day to complete a total of 14 days of therapy
- When tuboovarian abscess is present, many healthcare providers use clindamycin for continued therapy rather than doxycycline because clindamycin provides more effective anaerobic coverage
- **PID, Alternative Parenteral Regimens:** Limited data support the use of other parenteral regimens, but the following three regimens have been investigated in at least one clinical trial, and they have broad-spectrum coverage.

Ofloxacin............................. 400 mg IV every 12 hours, PLUS metronidazole 500 mg IV every 8 hours **OR**

Ampicillin/Sulbactam............ 3 g IV every 6 hours, PLUS doxycycline 100 mg IV / orally every 12 hours **OR**

Ciprofloxacin........................200 mg IV every 12 hours, PLUS doxycycline 100 mg IV or orally every 12 hours, **PLUS**

Metronidazole........................500 mg IV every 8 hours.

Oral Treatment: The following regimens provide coverage against the frequent etiologic agents of PID, but evidence from clinical trials supporting their use is limited. Patients who do not respond to oral therapy within 72 hours should be reevaluated to confirm the diagnosis and be administered parenteral therapy on either an outpatient or inpatient basis.

- **PID, Oral Regimen A**

Ofloxacin............................. 400 mg orally twice a day for 14 days, **PLUS**

Metronidazole........................500 mg orally twice a day for 14 days.

- **PID, Oral Regimen B**

Ceftriaxone............................250 mg IM once, **OR**

Cefoxitin................................2 g IM plus probenecid, 1 g orally in a single dose concurrently once, **OR**

Other parenteral third-generation cephalosporin (e.g.,ceftizoxime or cefotaxime), **PLUS**

Doxycycline........................ 100 mg orally twice a day for 14 days.

Follow-up:

- Patients receiving oral or parenteral therapy should demonstrate substantial clinical improvement (i.e., defervescence; reduction in direct or rebound abdominal tenderness; and reduction in uterine, adnexal, and cervical motion tenderness) within 3 days after initiation of therapy
- Patients who do not improve within 3 days usually require additional diagnostic tests, surgical intervention, or both
- If the health-care provider prescribes outpatient oral or parenteral therapy, a follow-up examination should be performed within 72 hours

Special Considerations:

- **Pregnancy:** Pregnant women who have suspected PID should be hospitalized and treated with parenteral antibiotics.

Genital Warts

- More than 20 types of HPV can infect the genital tract. Most HPV infections are asymptomatic, subclinical, or unrecognized. Visible genital warts usually are caused by HPV types 6 or 11. Other HPV types in the anogenital region (i.e., types 16, 18, 31, 33, and 35) have been strongly associated with cervical dysplasia
- No data support the use of type-specific HPV nucleic acid tests in the routine diagnosis or management of visible genital warts
- HPV types 6 and 11 also can cause warts on the uterine cervix and in the vagina, urethra and anus; these warts are sometimes symptomatic
- HPV types 6 and 11 are associated rarely with invasive squamous cell carcinoma of the external genitalia
- HPV types 16, 18, 31, 33, and 35 are found occasionally in visible genital warts and have been associated with external genital (i.e., vulvar, penile, and anal) squamous intraepithelial neoplasia (i.e., squamous cell carcinoma in situ, bowenoid papulosis, erythroplasia of Queyrat, or Bowen's disease of the genitalia). These HPV types have been associated with vaginal, anal, and cervical intraepithelial dysplasia and squamous cell carcinoma. Patients who have visible genital warts can be infected simultaneously with multiple HPV types

Treatment:

- The primary goal of treating visible genital warts is the removal of symptomatic warts
- Treatment can induce wart-free periods in most patients. Genital warts often are asymptomatic
- **No evidence indicates that currently available treatments eradicate or affect the natural history of HPV infection.** The removal of warts may or may not decrease infectivity
- If left untreated, visible genital warts may resolve on their own, remain unchanged, or increase in size or number. No evidence indicates that treatment of visible warts affects the development of cervical cancer

Regimens:

- Treatment of genital warts should be guided by the patient's preference, the available resources, and the experience of the health-care provider.
- None of the available treatments is superior to other treatments, and no single treatment is ideal for all circumstances. The treatment modality should be changed if a patient has not improved substantially after three provider-administered treatments or if warts have not completely cleared after six treatments
- Providers should be knowledgeable about, and have available, at least one patient-applied and one provider-administered treatment

- **External Genital Warts, Recommended Treatments:**
- *Patient-Applied*
Podofilox..................................0.5% solution or gel.
- Patients may apply podofilox solution with a cotton swab, or podofilox gel with a finger, to visible genital warts twice a day for 3 days, followed by 4 days of no therapy
- This cycle may be repeated as necessary for a total of four cycles
- The total wart area treated should not exceed 10 cm², and a total volume of podofilox should not exceed 0.5 mL per day
- If possible, the health-care provider should apply the initial treatment to demonstrate the proper application technique and identify which warts should be treated. The safety

of podofilox during pregnancy has not been established. **OR**

Imiquimod...........................5% cream.

- Patients should apply imiquimod cream with a finger at bedtime, three times a week for as long as 16 weeks
- The treatment area should be washed with mild soap and water 6-10 hours after the application
- Many patients may be clear of warts by 8-10 weeks or sooner
- The safety of imiquimod during pregnancy has not been established

- **Provider-Administered:**

Cryotherapy with liquid nitrogen or cryoprobe. Repeat applications every 1 to 2 weeks. **OR**

Podophyllin resin...................10%-25% in tincture of benzoin.

- A small amount should be applied to each wart and allowed to air dry
- To avoid the possibility of complications associated with systemic absorption and toxicity, some experts recommend that application be limited to <0.5 mL of podophyllin or <10 cm² of warts per session
- Some experts suggest that the preparation should be thoroughly washed off 1-4 hours after application to reduce local irritation. Repeat weekly if necessary
- *The safety of podophyllin during pregnancy has not been established* **OR**

TCA or BCA 80%-90%. May place petroleum jelly around wart to reduce spread of medication to normal mucosa. Apply a small amount only to warts and allow to dry, at which time a white "frosting" develops; powder with talc or NaHCO₃ to remove unreacted acid if an excess amount is applied. Repeat weekly if necessary. **OR**

- *Surgical removal* by tangential scissor excision, tangential shave excision, curettage, or electrosurgery

- **External Genital Warts, Alternative Treatments (Provider administered)**

Intra-lesional interferon **OR**

Laser surgery

- **Cervical Warts**

For women who have exophytic cervical warts, high-grade squamous intraepithelial lesions (SIL) must be excluded before treatment is begun. Management of exophytic cervical warts should include consultation with an expert

- **Vaginal Warts, Recommended Treatment**

Cryotherapy with liquid nitrogen. The use of a cryoprobe in the vagina is not recommended because of the risk for vaginal perforation and fistula formation. **OR**

TCA or BCA 80%-90% applied only to warts. Repeat weekly if necessary. **OR**

Podophyllin 10%-25% in compound tincture of benzoin applied to a treated area that must be dry before the speculum is removed. Repeat application at weekly intervals. The safety of podophyllin during pregnancy has not been established.

- **Urethral Meatus Warts, Recommended Treatment**

Cryotherapy with liquid nitrogen **OR**

Podophyllin 10%-25% in tincture of benzoin. The treatment area must be dry before contact with normal mucosa. Podophyllin must be applied weekly if necessary. *The safety of podophyllin during pregnancy has not been established.*

- **Anal Warts, Recommended Treatment**

Cryotherapy with liquid nitrogen **OR**

TCA or BCA 80%-90% applied to warts. Apply a small amount only to warts and allow to dry, at which time a white "frosting" develops; powder with talc or sodium bicarbonate (i.e., baking soda) to remove unreacted acid if an excess amount is applied. Repeat weekly if necessary. May place petroleum jelly around wart to reduce spread of medication to normal mucosa **OR**

Surgical removal

- Management of warts on rectal mucosa should be referred to an expert

Follow-up: After visible genital warts have cleared, a follow-up is not mandatory

Management of Sex Partners: None. Examination of sex partners is not necessary for the management of genital warts because the role of reinfection is probably minimal and, in the absence of curative therapy, treatment to reduce transmission is not realistic

Special Considerations:

- *Pregnancy:* Imiquimod, podophyllin, and podofilox should not be used during pregnancy. Because genital warts can proliferate and become friable during pregnancy, many experts advocate their removal during pregnancy. HPV types 6 and 11 can cause laryngeal papillomatosis in infants and children. Vaginal delivery not contraindicated unless lesion size obstructive in labor (rare). The route of transmission (i.e., transplacental, perinatal, or postnatal) is not completely understood

VACCINE-PREVENTABLE STIs

One of the most effective means of preventing the transmission of STIs is preexposure immunization. Currently licensed vaccines for the prevention of STIs include those for hepatitis A and hepatitis B. Clinical development and trials are underway for vaccines against a number of other STIs, including HIV and HSV. As more vaccines become available, immunization possibly will become one of the most widespread methods used to prevent STIs

ECTOPARASITIC INFECTIONS

PEDICULOSIS PUBIS

Patients who have pediculosis pubis (i.e., pubic lice) usually seek medical attention because of pruritus. Such patients also usually notice lice or nits on their pubic hair

Treatment:

- **Pediculosis Pubis, Recommended Regimens**

Permethrin..........................1% creme rinse applied to affected areas and washed off after 10 minutes **OR**

Lindane...............................1% shampoo applied for 4 minutes to the affected area, and then thoroughly washed off. This regimen is not recommended for pregnant or lactating women or for children aged <2 yrs **OR**

Pyrethrins with piperonyl butoxide applied to the affected area and washed off after 10 minutes.

Other Management Considerations:

- The recommended regimens should not be applied to the eyes. Pediculosis of the eyelashes should be treated by applying occlusive ophthalmic ointment to the eyelid margins twice a day for 10 days
- Bedding and clothing should be decontaminated (either machine-washed and machine-dried using the heat cycle or drycleaned) or removed from body contact for at least 72 hrs
- Fumigation of living areas is not necessary

Follow-up: Patients should be evaluated after 1 week if symptoms persist. Retreatment may ~~b~~e necessary if lice are found or if eggs are observed at the hair~~/~~skin junction. Patients who ~~d~~o not respond to one of the recommended regimens should be retreated with an alternative ~~r~~egimen

Management of Sex Partners: Sex partners within the last month should be treated

Special Considerations:
- **Pregnancy:** Pregnant and lactating women should be treated with either permethrin or pyrethrins with piperonyl butoxide

SCABIES

Predominant symptoms is pruritus; sensitization takes several weeks to develop; pruritus might occur within 24 hours after a subsequent reinfestation

Scabies in adults may be sexually transmitted, although scabies in children usually is not

- **Scabies, Recommended Regimen**

Permethrin cream.................(5%) applied to all areas of the body from the neck down and washed off after 8-14 hours.

- **Scabies, Alternative Regimens**

Lindane.................................(1%) 1 oz. of lotion or 30 g of cream applied thinly to all areas of the body from the neck down and thoroughly washed off after 8 hours **OR**

Sulfur...................................(6%) precipitated in ointment applied thinly to all areas nightly for 3 nights. Previous applications should be washed off before new applications are applied. Thoroughly wash off 24 hours after the last application.

- Lindane should not be used immediately after a bath, and it should not be used by a) persons who have extensive dermatitis, b) pregnant or lactating women, and c) children aged <2 years.

Other Management Considerations: Bedding and clothing should be decontaminated ~~(~~i.e., either machine-washed or machine-dried using the hot cycle or dry-cleaned) or ~~r~~emoved from body contact for at least 72 hours. Fumigation of living areas is unnecessary

Follow-up: Pruritus may persist for several weeks. Some experts recommend retreatment ~~a~~fter 1 week for patients who are still symptomatic; other experts recommend retreatment ~~o~~nly if live mites are observed. Patients who do not respond should be retreated with an ~~a~~lternative regimen

Management of Sex Partners and Household Contacts: Both sexual and close personal ~~o~~r household contacts within the preceding month should be examined and treated

SEXUAL ASSAULT AND STIs: Adults and Adolescents

Evaluation for Sexually Transmitted Infections
- **Initial Examination** - (See inside back cover)
- **Follow-up Examination after Assault**
  - Examination for STIs should be repeated 2 weeks after assault (see inside back cover)
  - Serologic tests for syphilis and HIV should be repeated 6, 12, and 24 weeks after the assault if initial test results were negative
- **Prophylaxis:** Many experts recommend routine preventive therapy after a sexual assault. The prophylactic regimen suggested is on inside back cover
- An empiric antimicrobial regimen for chlamydia, gonorrhea, trichomonas, and BV should be administered (See inside back cover)

Other Management Considerations:

At the initial examination and, if indicated, at follow-up, patients should be counseled about

- Risk for pregnancy and possible use of emergency contraception
- Symptoms of STIs and the need for immediate examination if symptoms occur
- Abstinence from sexual intercourse until STI prophylactic treatment is completed

Risk for Acquiring HIV Infection:

- Although HIV antibody seroconversion has been reported among persons whose only known risk factor was sexual assault or sexual abuse, the risk for acquiring HIV infection through sexual assault is low and depends on many factors
- These factors may include the type of sexual intercourse (i.e., oral, vaginal, or anal); presence of oral, vaginal or anal trauma; site of exposure to ejaculate; viral load in ejaculate; and presence of an STI

HIV INFECTION

This section has been adapted. For entire guidelines see www.cdc.gov/nchstp/dstd/ Proper management of HIV infection involves a complex array of behavioral, pyschosocial, and medical services. This information should not be a substitute for referral to a health-care provider or facility experienced in caring for HIV-infected patients. The following hotlines may provide excellent information and referrals for provider and patient:

CDC AIDS Treatment Information Service..........1-800-HIV-0440 (1-800-448-0440)
    e-mail to: atis@hivatis.org & www.hivatis.org
CDC AIDS Clinical Trials Information Service...1-800-TRIALS-A (1-800-874-2572)
    e-mailto: actis@actis.org
    International.............1-301-519-0459
For general information and referrals to local facilities:
CDC National AIDS Hotline.................................1-800-342-AIDS (1-800-342-2437)
    Spanish.............1-800-344-7432
CDC National AIDS Clearinghouse.......................1-800-458-5231
CDC Division of HIV/AIDS Prevention.................www.cdc.gov/hiv
Post exposure prophylaxis PEP............................1-888-HIV-4911

Pregnancy: All pregnant women should be offered HIV testing as early in pregnancy as possible. This recommendation is particularly important because of the available treatments for reducing the likelihood of perinatal transmission and maintaining the health of the woman. HIV-infected women should be informed specifically about the risk for perinatal infection. Current evidence indicates that 15%-25% of infants born to untreated HIV-infected mothers are infected with HIV; the virus also can be transmitted from an infected mother by breastfeeding. Zidovudine (ZDV) reduces the risk for HIV transmission to the infant from approximately 25% to 8% if administered to women during the later stage of pregnancy and during labor and to infants for the first 6 weeks of life. Therefore, **ZDV TREATMENT SHOULD BE OFFERED TO ALL HIV-INFECTED PREGNANT WOMEN**. Most women in the U.S. now receive triple therapy during pregnancy not just ZDV. In the United States, HIV-infected women should be advised not to breast-feed their infants. In other countries, the reduced risk of death from malnutrition, diarrheal disease, or other infections may outweigh the risk of contracting HIV.

Insufficient information is available regarding the safety of ZDV or other antiretroviral drugs during early pregnancy; however, on the basis of the ACTG-076 protocol, ZDV is indicated for the prevention of maternal-fetal HIV transmission as part of a regimen that includes oral ZDV at 14-34 weeks of gestation, intravenous (IV) ZDV during labor, and ZDV syrup to the neonate after birth.

WHO MEDICAL ELIGIBILITY CRITERIA FOR STARTING CONTRACEPTIVE METHODS (2001) ◄─

The table on the following pages summarizes the latest World Health Organization (WHO) medical eligibility criteria for starting contraceptives. These criteria are also the basis for the checklists throughout *Managing Contraception*. These criteria are for the most part evidence-based. References are available through the World Health Organization

WHO categories for temporary methods:

WHO 1   **Can use** the method. No restriction on use.

WHO 2   **Can use** the method. Advantages generally outweigh theoretical or proven risks. If method is chosen, more than usual follow-up may be needed.

WHO 3   **Should not use** the method unless clinician makes clinical judgment that the patient can safely use it. **Theoretical or proven risks usually outweigh the advantages** of method. Method of last choice, for which regular monitoring may be needed.

WHO 4   **Should not use** the method. Condition represents an unacceptable health risk if method is used.

Simplified 2-category system for temporary methods

To make clinical judgment, the WHO 4-category classification system can be simplified into a 2-category system.

WHO Category	With Clinical Judgment	With Limited Clinical Judgment
1	Use the method in any circumstances	Use the method
2	Generally use the method	Use the method
3	Use of the method not usually recommended unless other, more appropriate methods are not available or acceptable	Do not use the method
4	Method not to be used	Do not use the method

NOTE: In the pages that follow, Category 3 and 4 conditions are shaded to indicate the method should not be provided where clinical judgment is limited.

A1

WHO MEDICAL ELIGIBILITY CRITERIA FOR STARTING CONTRACEPTIVE METHODS (2001)

CONDITION	Combined OCs	Combined Injectables	Progestin-Only OCs	Depo-Provera NET EN	Norplant Implants	Condoms	Spermicides	Diaphragm	TCu-380A IUD	LNG IUD
PERSONAL CHARACTERISTICS & REPRODUCTIVE HISTORY										
Pregnant	NA	NA	NA	NA	NA	NA	NA	NA	4	4
Age	Menarche to <40=1 / ≥40=2	Menarche to <40=1 / ≥40=2	Menarche to <18=1 / 18-45=1 / >45=1	Menarche to <18=2 / 18-45=1 / >45=2	Menarche to <40=1 / 18-45=1 / >45=1	Menarche to <40=1 / ≥40=1	Menarche to <40=1 / ≥40=1	Menarche to <40=1 / ≥40=1	<20=2 / ≥20=1	<20=2 / ≥20=1
Parity a) nulliparous	1	1	1	1	1	1	1	1	2	2
b) parous	1	1	1	1	1	1	1	1	1	1
Breastfeeding < 6 weeks PP	4	4	3	3	3					
≥ 6 weeks to 6 months PP primarily breastfeeding	3	3	1	1	1					
≥ 6 months PP	2	2	1	1	1					
Postpartum < 21 days	3	3	1	1	1				<48 hrs 1 / 48h-<4wks 3 / ≥4 wks 1	<48 hrs 3 / 48h-<4wks 3 / >4 wks 4
≥ 21 days	1		1	1	1					
Puerperal Sepsis									4	4
Post-abortion 1st trimester	1	1	1	1	1	1	1	1	1	1
2nd trimester	1	1	1	1	1	1	1	1	2	2
Immediate post septic AB	1	1	1	1	1	1	1	1	4	4
Past ectopic pregnancy	1	1	2	1	1	1	1	1	1	1

For women greater than 45 there are concerns regarding hypo-estrogenic effect of DMPA on bone mass.

There is concern that the neonate may be at risk of exposure to steroid hormones during the first 6 weeks. POCs may be one of the few types methods available and accessible to breastfeeding women immediately postpartum.

A2

When multiple major risk factors exist, risk of CV disease may increase substantially. Some POCs may increase risk of thrombosis although this risk is substantially less than with COCs.

History of pelvic surgery	1	1	1	1	1	1
Smoking: Less than age 35	2	2	1	1	1	1
Age ≥ 35 < 15 cigarettes/day	3	2	1	1	1	1
Age ≥ 35 ≥ 15 cigarettes/day	4	3	1	1	1	1
Obesity ≥ 30 kg/m² BMI	2	2	2	1	1	2
CARDIOVASCULAR DISEASE						
Multiple risk factors for CAD (older age, smoking, diabetes, HBP)	3 or 4	3 or 4	2	3	1	2
HBP Hx HBP; BP can't be evaluated	3	3	2	2	1	2
HBP adequately controlled	3	3	1	2	1	1
BP systolic 140-159 or Diastolic 90-99	3	3	2	1	1	1
BP systolic > 160 or Diastolic 100	4	4	3	3	1	2
Vascular disease	4	4	2	3	1	2
HBP during pregnancy, BP now normal	2	2	1	1	1	1
Deep vein thrombosis/pulmonary embolism						
a) History of DVT/PE	4	4	2	2	1	2
b) Current DVT/PE	4	4	3	3	1	3
c) Family History (first-degree relatives)	2	2	1	1	1	1
d) Major surgery with prolonged immobilization	4	4	2	2	1	2
e) Major surgery without prolonged immobilization	2	2	1	1	1	1
f) Minor surgery without immobilization	1	1	1	1	1	1

A3

WHO MEDICAL ELIGIBILITY CRITERIA FOR STARTING CONTRACEPTIVE METHODS (CONTINUED)

CONDITION	Combined OCs	Combined Injectables	Progestin-Only OCs	Depo-Provera NET EN	Norplant Implants	Condoms	Spermicides	Diaphragm	TCu-380A IUD	LNG IUD
Superficial venous thrombosis										
a) varicose veins	1	1	1	1	1	1	1	1	1	1
b) superficial thrombophlebitis	2	2	1	1	1	1	1	1	1	1
Current & history of ischemic heart disease	4	4	2/3*	3	2/3	1	1	1	1	2/3
Stroke (history of CVA)	4	4	2/3	3	2/3	1	1	1	1	2
Known hyperlipidemia	2* or 3	2 or 3	2	2	2	1	1	1	2	2
Valvular heart disease uncomplicated	2	2	1	1	1	1	1	1	1	1
Valvular heart disease complicated	4	4	1	1	1	1	1	1	2	2
NEUROLOGIC CONDITIONS										
Headaches										
a) non-migraine (mild or severe)	1/2	1/2	1/1	1/1	1/1	1	1	1	1/1	1/1
b) migraine < 35; no focal neurologic symptoms	2/3	2/3	1/2	2/2	2/2	1	1	1	2/2	2/2
c) migraine ≥ 35; no focal neurologic symptoms	3/4	3/4	1/2	2/2	2/2	1	1	1	2/2	2/2
d) migraine with focal neurologic Sx (any age)	4/4	4/4	2/3	2/3	2/3	1	1	1	2/2	2/2
Epilepsy	1	1	1	1	1	1	1	1	1	1
REPRODUCTIVE TRACT INFECTIONS & DISORDERS										
Irregular without heavy bleeding	1	1	2	2	2	1	1	1	1	1/1
Heavy or prolonged vaginal bleeding (regular or irregular)	1	1	2	2	2	1	1	1	2	1/2
Unexplained vaginal bleeding. Suspicious for serious underlying condition. Before evaluation	2	2	2	3	2	1	1	1	4/2	4/2

* Initiation: 2 and Continuation: 3 expressed as 2/3 (I/C)

** If distinction is made between levels of severity it is expressed as 2 or 3

Margin notes:

→ Varicose Veins are not risk factors for DVT/PE

→ There is concern regarding reduced HDL levels among POC users. Some POQs may increase the risk of arterial thrombosis, although this increase is substantially less than with COCs.

→ New evidence: Among women with migraines, women who also have focal neurologic symptoms have a higher risk of stroke than those without focal neurologic symptoms. In addition, among women with migraines, those who use COCs have a 2 to 4-fold increased risk of stroke compared with women who do not use COCs.

A4

Condition										
Endometriosis	1	1	1	1	1	1	1	1	2	1
Benign ovarian tumors (including cysts)	1	1	1	1	1	1	1	1	1	1
Severe dysmenorrhea	1	1	1	1	1	1	1	1	2	1
Benign gestational trophoblastic disease	1	1	1	1	1	1	1	1	3	3
Malignant gestational trophoblastic disease	1	1	1	1	1	1	1	1	4	4
Cervical ectropion	1	1	1	1	1	1	1	1	1	1
Cervical intraepithelial neoplasia (CIN)	2	2	1	2	2	1	1	1	2	2
Cervical cancer (awaiting treatment)	2	2	1	2	2	1	2	1	4*/2	4/2
Undiagnosed breast mass	2	2	2	2	2	1	1	1	2	
Benign breast disease	1	1	1	1	1	1	1	1	1	
Family history of breast cancer	1	1	1	1	1	1	1	1	1	
Breast cancer (current)	4	4	4	4	4	1	1	1	4	
Past breast cancer: No current disease for 5 years	3	3	3	3	3	1	1	1	3	
Endometrial cancer	1	1	1	1	1	1	1	1	4/2	4/2
Ovarian cancer	1	1	1	1	1	1	1	1	3/2	3/2
Uterine fibroids *without* distortion of uterine cavity	1	1	1	1	1	1	1	1	2	2
Uterine fibroids *with* distortion of uterine cavity	1	1	1	1	1	1	1	1	4	4

Copper IUD may worsen dysmenorrhea associated with endometriosis

There is some concern that COCs enhance the progression of CIN to invasive disease, particularly with long-term use

Breast cancer is hormonally sensitive, and the prognosis of women with current or recent breast cancer may worsen with COC or POC use

WHO MEDICAL ELIGIBILITY CRITERIA FOR STARTING CONTRACEPTIVE METHODS (CONTINUED)

CONDITION	Combined OCs	Combined Injectables	Progestogen-Only OCs	Depo-Provera NET EN	Norplant Implants	Condoms	Spermicides	Diaphragm	Tcu-380A IUD	LNG IUD	
Past history PID (no current STI risk factors) with subsequent pregnancy	1	1	1	1	1	1	1	1	1/1	1/1	
Past history PID (no current STI risk factors) without subsequent pregnancy	1	1	1	1	1	1	1	1	2/2	2/2	In women at low risk of STIs, IUD insertion poses little risk of PID. Current risk of STIs and desire for future pregnancy are relevant considerations
Current PID (or within last 3 months)	1	1	1	1	1	1	1	1	4/3	4/3	
STI: current or past 3 months (including purulent cervicitis)	1	1	1	1	1	1	1	1	4	4	
Vaginitis without purulent cervicitis	1	1	1	1	1	1	1	1	2	2	
Increased risk of STIs	1	1	1	1	1	1	1	1	3	3	
HIV/AIDS											
High risk of HIV	1	1	1	1	1	2	1	1	3	3	Women at high risk of HIV are also at high risk of toher STIs
HIV-positive	1	1	1	1	1	2	1	1	3	3	
AIDS	1	1	1	1	1	2	1	1	3	3	
ENDOCRINE CONDITIONS											
History gestational diabetes	1	1	1	1	1	1	1	1	1	1	
Non-insulin dependent diabetes (non-vascular disease)	2	2	2	2	2	1	1	1	1	2	
Insulin dependent diabetes (non-vascular disease)	2	2	2	2	2	1	1	1	1	2	
Diabetic nephropathy/retinopathy/neuropathy	3/4	3/4	2	3	2	1	1	1	1	2	There is concern about the possible negative effect of DMPA on lipid metabolism, possibly affecting the progression of nephropathy, retopa-
Other vascular disease, diabetes of > 20 years	3/4	3/4	2	3	2	1	1	1	1	2	

* Initiation: 4 and Continuation: 3 expressed as 4/3 (IUC)

Condition									Notes
Thyroid: simple goiter	1	1	1	1	1	1	1	1	
Hyperthyroid	1	1	1	1	1	1	1	1	
Hypothyroid	1	1	1	1	1	1	1	1	
GASTROINTESTINAL CONDITIONS									
Symptomatic gall bladder disease post cholecystectomy	2	2	2	2	1	1	1	2	COCs may cause small increased risk of gall bladder disease. There is also concern that COCs may worsen existing gall-bladder disease
Symptomatic gall bladder disease medically treated	3	2	2	2	1	1	1	2	
Symptomatic gall bladder disease - current	3	2	2	2	1	1	1	2	
Asymptomatic gall bladder disease	2	2	2	2	1	1	1	2	
History of pregnancy-related cholestasis	2	1	1	1	1	1	1	2	
Past COC-related cholestasis	3	2	2	2	1	1	1	2	
Viral hepatitis active	4	3/4*	3	3	1	1	1	3	COCs are metabolized by liver and use may adversely affect women whose liver function is already compromised. There is concern about the hormonal load associated with POC use, but it is less than for COCs
Viral hepatitis carrier	1	1	1	1	1	1	1	1	
Cirrhosis: mild compensated	3	2	2	2	1	1	1	2	
Benign hepatic adenoma	4	3	3	3	1	1	1	3	
Malignant liver tumor (hepatoma)	4	3/4	3	3	1	1	1	3	

*Initiation: 3 and Continuation: 4 expressed as 3/4 (I/C)

WHO MEDICAL ELIGIBILITY CRITERIA FOR STARTING CONTRACEPTIVE METHODS (CONTINUED)

CONDITION	Combined OCs	Combined Injectables	Progestin-Only OCs	Depo-Provera NET EN	Norplant Implants	Condoms	Spermicides	Diaphragm	TCu-380A IUD	LNG IUD
ANEMIAS										
Thalassemia	1	1	1	1	1	1	1	1	2	1
Sickle cell disease	2	2	1	1	1	1	1	1	2	1
Iron deficiency anemia	1	1	1	1	1	1	1	1	2	1
DRUG INTERACTIONS										
Rifampicine & griseofulvin	3	3	3	2	3	1	1	1	1	1
Anticonvulsants: Phenytoin, barbiturates carbamazepine, primadone	3	3	3	2	3	1	1	1	1	1
Other antibiotics (other than rifampicin/griseofulvin)	1	1	1	1	NA	1	1	1	1	1
Allergy to latex	NA	NA	NA	NA	NA	3	1	3	NA	NA

← ← Although the interaction between commonly used liver enzyme inducers and COGs is not harmful to women, it is likely to reduce the efficacy of COGs. Use of other contraceptives should be encouraged for women who are long-term users of any of these drugs. Whether increasing the hormone dose of COGs is of benefit remains unclear.

HISTORY OF CONTRACEPTION AND POPULATION GROWTH

"We have not inherited the earth from our grandparents, we have borrowed it from our grandchildren."
—Professor John Guillebaud-Attributed to the Ancient Chinese

2000	RU486 (mifepristone), Lunelle and Mirena approved by FDA
1999	World population hits **6 billion** (this billion took 12 years)
1997	FDA approves Emergency Contraceptive Pills
1994	Plastic (polyurethane) condom for men (Avanti)
1993	FDA approves polyurethane (plastic) female condom (Reality)
1993	Creinin and Darney describe medical abortion using methotrexate
1992	FDA approves Depo-Provera (DMPA) injections
1990	FDA approves Norplant implants
1988	Copper T 380-A IUD marketing begins, 5 years after FDA approval
1987	World population reaches **5 billion** (this billion took 12 years)
1983	FDA approves Copper T 380-A and the Today sponge
1982	Baulieu describes medical abortion using mifepristone
1981	First case of HIV/AIDS
1981	Garret Hardin writes "nobody ever dies of overpopulation" after 500,000 die from flooding of an overcrowded East Bengal River delta
1975	World population reaches **4 billion** (this billion took 15 years)
1974	Al Yuzpe describes emergency contraception using Ovral pills
1973	FDA approves progestin-only pills (minipills)
1973	U.S. Supreme Court abortion decision (Roe v Wade & Doe v Bolton)
1965	U.S. Supreme Court Griswold v. CT, overturns anti-birth control laws in most states
1965	U.S. Agency of International Development initiates Population Program
1960	Food and Drug Administration approves combined oral contraceptives
1960	World population reaches **3 billion** (this billion took 30 years)
1942	American Birth Control League renamed Planned Parenthood
1937	AMA ends longstanding opposition to contraception
1936	German gynecologist Friedrich Wilde describes first cervical cap (fitted from a wax impression)
1930-31	Knaus (Austria) and Ogino (Japan) develop rhythm method
1930	World population now **2 billion** (this billion took 100 years)
1930	Pope Pius XI virulently attacks both contraception & abortion
1927	Novak (Hopkins) describes suction as means of performing an abortion
1916	Margaret Sanger opens first Amercian birth control clinic in Brooklyn, NY
1914	Margaret Sanger coins word "birth control"
1912	Sadie Sachs post-abortion death affects Margaret Sanger profoundly
1909	German surgeon Richard Richter reports success with silkworm-gut shaped into a ring
1904	Basal body temperature fluctuations described
1893	First vasectomy by Harrison in London
1882	First contraceptive clinic established in Amsterdam
1880	First tubal ligation
1873	Comstock Act: classifies all images on contraception as obscene
1839	Charles Goodyear discovers vulcanization technology; quickly leads to rubber condoms
1830	World population reaches **1 billion** (this billion took 6 million years)
1798	Thomas Robert Malthus proposes dismal economic theory that a population growth eventually will exceed the ability of the earth to provide food, resulting in starvation
Late 1770s	Casanova popularizes condoms for infection control and contraception
1 AD	World population reaches **250 million**, abstinence (particularly postpartum), withdrawal, lactation, stones in camels, lemons for mechanical and spermicidal effect, abortion using molokeeia (same root used today), homosexuality and polygamy

Timeline annotations:
- 1999 - 6 billion (10/12/99!!)
- 1987 - 5 billion
- 1975 - 4 billion
- 1960 - 3 billion
- 1930 - 2 billion
- 1800 - 1 billion
- 1 AD - 250 million

Special thanks to Andrea Tone at Georgia Tech

American College of Obstetrics and Gynecologists (ACOG). Emergency oral contraception. ACOG Practice Patterns 1996 (Dec. no. 3).

Berel V, Hermon C, Kay C, Hannaford P, Darby S, Reeves G. Mortality associated with oral contraceptive use: 25 year follow-up of cohort of 46,000 women from Royal College of General Practitioners' oral contraceptive study; Br Med J 1999: 918:96-100.

Brache V, Alvarez-Sanchez F, Faundes A, Tejada AS, Cochon L. Ovarian endocrine function through five years of continuous treatment with Norplant subdermal contraceptive implants. Contraception 1990;41:169.

Briggs GG, Freeman RK, Yaffe SJ. Drugs in Pregnancy and Lactation, Fifth edition. Lippincott Williams & Wilkins, Philadelphia. 1998.

Centers for Disease Control and Prevention. 1998 Guidelines for treatment of sexually transmitted diseases. MMWR 1998;47(No. RR-1): 1-118

Creinin MD, Burke AE. Methotrexate and misoprostol for early abortion: a multicenter trial. Acceptablity. Contraception 1996;54:19-22.

Creinin MD, Vittinghoff E, Schaff E, Klaisle C, Darney PD, Dean C. Medical abortion with oral methotrexate and vaginal misoprostol. Obstet Gynecol 1997;90:611-5.

Cromer BA, Blair JM, Mahan JD, Zibners L, Naumovski Z. A prospective comparison of bone density in adolescent girls receiving depo-medroxyprogesteroneacetate (Depo-Provera), levonorgestrel (Norplant), or oral contraceptives. J Pediatr 1996;129:671-6.

Croxatto HB, Diaz S, Pavez M, et al. Plasma progesterone levels during long-term treatment with levonorgestrel silastic implants. Acta Endocrinol 1982;101:307-11.

Farley TM, Rosenberg MS, Rowe PJ, Chen SH, Meirck O. Intrauterine devices and pelvic inflammatory disease: an international perspective. Lancet 1992; 339: 785-88.

Feldblum PJ, Morrison CS, Roddy RE, Cates W Jr. The effectiveness of barrier methods of contraception in preventing the spread of HIV. AIDS 1995;9 (suppl A):585-93.

Fraser SI, Affandi B, Croxatto HB, et al. Norplant consensus statement and background paper. Turku, Finland: Leiras Oy International, 1997.

Frezieres RG, Walsh TL, Nelson AL, Clark VA, Coulson AH: Breakage and acceptability of a polyurethane condom: A randomized controlled study. *Fam Plann Perspect* 1998;30;73-8

Goldstein M, Girardi S. Vasectomy and vasectomy reversal. Curr Thera Endocrinol Metab 1997;6:371-80.

Gray RH, Campbell OM, Zacur H, Labbok MH, MacRae SL. Postpartum return of ovarian activity in non-breastfeeding women monitored by urinary assays. J Clin Endocrinol Metab 1987;64:645-50.

Grimes DA. Modern IUDs: an update. The Contraception Report; November, 1998

Guillebaud J. Contraception, your questions answered, 3rd edition. London, Churchill Livingstone, 1999.

Hafner DW, Schwartz P. What I've Learned about Sex. A Perigee Book: New York: The Berkeley Publishing Group, 1998.

Hakim-Elahi E, Tovell HMM, Burnhill MS. Complications of first-trimester abortion: a report of 170,000 cases. Obstet Gynecol 1990;76:129.

Henshaw SK. Unintended pregnancy in the United States. Fam Plann Perspect 1998;30:24-9, 46.

Hatcher RA, Trussell J, Stewart F, Cates W Jr, Stewart GK, Guest F, Kowal D. *Contraceptive Technology*, 17th ed. New York NY, Ardent Media, 1998

Hogue CJR, Cates W Jr, Tietze C. The effects of induced abortion on subsequent reproduction. The Johns Hopkins University School of Hygiene and Public Health. Epidemiol Rev 1982;4:66 International Planned Parenthood Federation Handbook 1997.

A10   Kaunitz AM. personal communication; December 28, 1998 and February 24, 1999.

Kennedy KI, Trussel J. Postpartum contraception and lactation. IN Hatcher RA, Trussell J, Stewart F et al: Contraceptive Technology, 17th ed.; New York: Ardent Media Inc; 1998: 592-4. [The same data are presented in the Family Health International Module for the teaching of Lactational Amenorrhea]

Kjos SL, Peters RK, Xiang A, Duncan T, Schaefer U, Buchanan TA. Contraception and the risk of type 2 diabetes mellitus in Latina women with prior gestational diabetes mellitus. JAMA 1998; 280: 533-38.

Klavon SL, Grubb G. Insertion site complications during the first year of Norplant use. Contraception 1990;41:27.

Miller L, Grice J. Intradermal proximal field block: an innovative anesthetic technique for levonorgestrel implant removal. *Obstet Gynecol* 1998;91:294-7

Narod ST. The Hereditary Cancer Clinical Study Group. Oral contraceptives and the risk of hereditary ovarian cancer. N Engl J Med 1998;339;424-8.

Peipert JF, Gutman J. Oral contraceptive risk assessment: a survey of 247 educated women. Obstet Gynecol 1993;82:112-7.

Peterson HB, Jeng G, Folger SG et al for the U.S. Collaborative Review of Sterilization Working Group. N Engl J Med 2000; 343:1681-7.

Peterson HB, Pollack AE, Warshaw JS. Tubal sterilization. In: Rock JA, Thompson JD, eds. TeLinde's Operative Gynecology. 8th ed. Philadelphia: Lippincott-Raven, 1997:541-5.

Raudaskoski TH, Lahti EI, Kauppila AJ, Apaja-Sarkkinen MA, Laatikainen TJ. Transdermal estrogen with a levonorgestrel-releasing intrauterine device for climacteric complaints: clinical and endometrial responses. Am J Obstet Gynecol 1995;172:114-9.

Redmond G, Godwin AJ, Olson W, Lippman JS. Use of placebo controls in an oral contraceptive trial: methodological issues and adverse event incidence. *Contraception* 1999;60:81-5.

The Alan Guttmacher Institute. Sex and America's Teenagers. New York and Washington: 1994.

Silvestre L, Dubois C, Renault M, Rezvani Y, Baulieu E, Ulmann A. Voluntary interruption of pregnancy with mifepristone (RU-486) and a prostaglandin analogue. N Engl J Med 1990; 322:645-8.

Smith TW. Personal communication to James Trussell. December 13, 1993.

Speroff L, Glass RH, Kase NG. Clinical Gynecologic Endocrinology and Infertility. Sixth Edition. 1999; Lipincott Williams & Wilkins; Baltimore, Maryland.

Speroff L. The perimenopausaual transition: maximizing preventive health care. In: Mooney B, Daughtery J, eds. Midlife Women's Health Sourcebook. Atlanta: American Health Consultants, 1995.

Task Force on Postovulatory Methods of Fertility Regulation. Randomized controlled trial of levonorgestrel versus the Yuzpe regimen of combined oral contraceptives for emergency contraception. Lancet 1998;352:420-33.

The Hereditary Ovarian Cancer Clinical Study Group. Oral contraceptives and the risk of hereditary ovarian cancer. N Engl J Med 1998;339;424-8.

Trussell J, Leveque JA, Koenig JD, et al. The economic value of contraception: a comparison of 15 methods. Am J Public Health 1995;85:494-503.

Trussell J, Stewart F, Guest F, Hatcher RA. Emergency contraceptive pills: a simple proposal to reduce unintended pregnancies. Fam Plann Perspect 1992;24:269-73.

Walsh T, Grimes D, Frezieres R, Nelson A, Bernstein L, Coulson A, Bernstein G. Randomized controlled trial of prophylactic antibiotics before insertion of intrauterine devices. *Lancet* 1998;351;1005-1008

White MK, Ory HW, Rooks JB, Rochat RW. Intrauterine device termination rates and menstrual cycle day of insertion. Obstet Gynecol 1980; 55:220-4.

World Health Organization. WHO Taskforce Postovulatory Methods of Fertility Regulation. Lancet Aug 8, 1998.

TOPIC	WEBSITE
Abortion	www.naral.org
	www.prochoice.org
Adolescent Reproductive Health	www.teenpregnancy.org
	www.ama-assn.org/adolhlth/adolhlth.htm
	www.advocatesforyouth.org
Contraception	www.conrad.org
	www.ippf.org
	www.plannedparenthood.org
	www.reproline.jhu.edu
	www.avsc.org/avsc
Counseling	www.gmhc.org
Education	www.siecus.org
	www.cdc.gov
Emergency Contraception	www.not-2-late.com (ec.princeton.edu)
HIV/AIDS/STIs	www.CritPath.Org/aric
	www.cdc.gov/hiv
	www.cdc.gov/nchstp/dstd/dstdp.htm
Managing Contraception	www.managingcontraception.com
Menopause	www.menopause.org
Natural Family Planning	www.canfp.org
	www.familyplanning.net
	www.ccli.org
Population Organizations	www.popcouncil.org
	www.prb.org
	www.undp.org/popin/infoserv.htm
	www.population.org/homepage.htm
Professional Organizations	www.acog.org
	www.arhp.org
	www.fda.gov
	www.fhi.org
	www.jsi.com
	www.obgyn.net
	www.pathfind.org
	www.plannedparenthood.org
	www.who.int
Reproductive Health Research	www.agi-usa.org
	www.kff.org
	www.fhi.org

SPANISH/ENGLISH TRANSLATIONS

SPANISH/ESPAÑOL

- Abstinencia
- Amamantar a Su Bebe
- Tapa Cervical
- Retraer el pene antes de ejecular
- Injecciones Combinadas
- La Pildora
- Condones parce hombres
- Condones para Mujeres
- La "T" o Dispositivo do Cobre
- Injecciones de Depo-Provera
- El Diafragma
- Contraceptivo de Emergencia
- Consciente Sobre Metodos de Fertilidad
- Espuma Contraceptiva
- Metodos para el Futuro
- Dispositivos
- Gelatina Anticonceptiva
- El Dispositivo de "Levo Norgestrel"
- Implantes de NORPLANT
- El Dispositivo de "Progestasert"
- Contraceptives de Progesterona Solamente
- Pildoras de Progesterona solamente
- RU-486 (Mifepristone)
- Espermicidas
- Ligadura o Estirilizacion de las Trompas
- Tela Anticonceptiva
- Vasectomia
- Todos los dispositivos

ENGLISH/INGLES

- Abstinence
- Breast-feeding
- Cervical Cap
- Coitus Interruptus (Withdrawal)
- Combined Injectables
- Combined Oral Contraceptives (COCs)
- Condoms for Men
- Condoms for Women
- Copper T 380-A
- Depo-Provera
- Diaphragm
- Emergency Contraception
- Fertility Awareness Methods
- Foam
- Future Methods
- IUDs
- Jellies
- Levonorgestrel IUD
- Norplant Implant
- Progestasert IUD
- Progestin-Only Contraceptives
- Progestin-Only Pills (POPs)
- RU-486 (Mifepristone)
- Spermicides
- Tubal Sterilization
- Vaginal contraceptive film
- Vasectomy
- All other IUDs at this time

<u>NOTE</u>: Final pages of Appendix (A14 - A22) are at very end of book

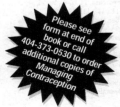

Please see form at end of book or call 404-373-0530 to order additional copies of Managing Contraception

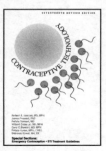

The Quest for Excellence

or high school students 13 to 18

he Quest for Excellence is a must for teaching
nd learning reproductive health. Deals with
How to Say No" and building self-esteem
round a healthy sexual identity. For teenagers
nd parents of teenagers.

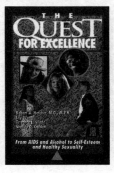

Size: 3.5" x 5.5"
182 pages

Sexual Etiquette 101 & More

For college students & all young adults (18-22)

ncludes current information on the following:

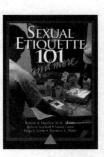

- Filled with actual case histories and many
  illustrations.
- Making a Personal Life Plan, Decision-Making
  Skills, Developing Self-Esteem, Learning to
  Communicate
- Your Body, The Menstrual Cycle, Expressing Your
  Sexuality, Masturbation, Sexual Concerns
- Sexually Transmitted Diseases: What are these
  and how to protect yourself against them.
- Contraception and Emergency Contraception

Size: 4.25" x 6.25"
160 pages

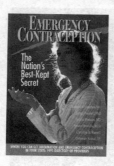
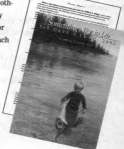

	Quantity	Total
Pocket Guide to Managing Contraception (for clinicians)		
10.00 ea	_____	_____
-199 9.00 ea	_____	_____
-299 8.00 ea	_____	_____
Guia de Bolsillo Para El Uso de Anticoncepion (Pocket Guide in Spanish)		
10.00 ea	_____	_____
-199 6.00 ea	_____	_____
-299 4.00 ea	_____	_____
or more 3.00 ea	_____	_____
Personal Guide to Managing Contraception for Women and Men (for the general public)		
14.95 ea	_____	_____
-199 11.95 ea	_____	_____
-299 10.95 ea	_____	_____
Contraceptive Technology - 17th Edition		
39.95 ea	_____	_____
0 35.00 ea	_____	_____
00 28.00 ea	_____	_____
Sexual Etiquette 101 & More		
4.95 ea	_____	_____
99 2.00 ea	_____	_____
-999 1.50 ea	_____	_____
0 up 1.00 ea	_____	_____
Quest for Excellence		
4.95 ea	_____	_____
99 2.00 ea	_____	_____
-999 1.50 ea	_____	_____
0 up 1.00 ea	_____	_____
Emergency Contraception (The Nation's Best Kept Secret)		
10.00 ea	_____	_____
Something Nice 2002 Calendar		
10.00 ea	_____	_____
499 8.00 ea	_____	_____
Emergency Contraceptive Kits		
minimum) 35.00 ea	_____	_____
00 3.00 ea	_____	_____
-500 2.50 ea	_____	_____
-1000 1.50 ea	_____	_____
Sub total		_____
Georgia locations add 7% sales tax		_____
Add $1.00 + 15% Shipping & Handling		_____
Total Enclosed		_____

accept check or credit cards: *VISA, MasterCard, Discover & American Express*

edit Card No. _____ Expiration Date: _____

nature: _____ –__ (Required)

IP TO: Name: _____

ganization: _____

ress: _____

_____ Zip _____

one No. _____ Fax No. _____

or Fax this ORDER FORM with your payment to:
ging the Gap Communications • P.O. Box 33218 • Decatur, GA 30033
e checks payable to Bridging the Gap Communications
ne: (404) 373-0530 • Fax: (404) 373-0480 • www.managingcontraception.com • email: savenow@projectplanetcorp.com

NK YOU! (CALL FOR SPECIAL PRICES ON LARGER QUANTITIES & INTERNATIONAL SHIPPING)   JS/RAH 4/01

		Quantity	Total
A Pocket Guide to Managing Contraception (for clinicians)			
1-99	10.00 ea	_____	_____
100-199	9.00 ea	_____	_____
200-299	8.00 ea	_____	_____
Una Guia de Bolsillo Para El Uso de Anticoncepcion (Pocket Guide in Spanish)			
1-99	10.00 ea	_____	_____
100-199	6.00 ea	_____	_____
200-299	4.00 ea	_____	_____
300 or more	3.00 ea	_____	_____
Personal Guide to Managing Contraception for Women and Men (for the general public)			
1-99	14.95 ea	_____	_____
100-199	11.95 ea	_____	_____
200-299	10.95 ea	_____	_____
Contraceptive Technology - 17th Edition			
1-24	39.95 ea	_____	_____
25-50	35.00 ea	_____	_____
51-100	28.00 ea	_____	_____
Sexual Etiquette 101 & More			
1-24	4.95 ea	_____	_____
25-499	2.00 ea	_____	_____
500-999	1.50 ea	_____	_____
1000 up	1.00 ea	_____	_____
Quest for Excellence			
1-24	4.95 ea	_____	_____
25-499	2.00 ea	_____	_____
500-999	1.50 ea	_____	_____
1000 up	1.00 ea	_____	_____
Emergency Contraception (The Nation's Best Kept Secret)			
1-99	10.00 ea	_____	_____
Something Nice 2002 Calendar			
1-9	10.00 ea	_____	_____
10-499	8.00 ea	_____	_____
Emergency Contraceptive Kits			
10 (minimum)	35.00 ea	_____	_____
11-100	3.00 ea	_____	_____
101-500	2.50 ea	_____	_____
501-1000	1.50 ea	_____	_____
	Sub total		_____
	Georgia locations add 7% sales tax		_____
	Add $1.00 + 15% Shipping & Handling		_____
	Total Enclosed		_____

We accept check or credit cards: VISA, MasterCard, Discover & American Express

Credit Card No. _____ Expiration Date: _____

Signature: _____ –__ (Requir

SHIP TO: Name: _____

Organization: _____

Address: _____

_____ Zip _____

Phone No. _____ Fax No. _____

Mail or Fax this ORDER FORM with your payment to:
Bridging the Gap Communications • P.O. Box 33218 • Decatur, GA 30033
Make checks payable to Bridging the Gap Communications
Phone: (404) 373-0530 • Fax: (404) 373-0480 • www.managingcontraception.com • email: savenow@projectplanetcorp.

THANK YOU! (CALL FOR SPECIAL PRICES ON LARGER QUANTITIES & INTERNATIONAL SHIPPING)

JS/RAI

OUR MISSION

The mission of *Bridging The Gap Foundation* is to improve reproductive health and contraceptive decision making of women and men by providing up-to-date educational resources to the health care providers of tomorrow.

OUR VISION

Our vision is to provide educational resources to the health care providers of tomorrow to help ensure informed choices, better service, access, happier and more successful contraceptors, competent clinicians, fewer unintended pregnancies and disease prevention.

www.managingcontraception.com

COLOR PHOTOS
of Combined and Progestin-Only Oral Contraceptives
www.managingcontraception.com ⬅

The eight color pages of pills are organized as follows:

* There are prominent horizontal or vertical parallel lines ("equal signs") between pills which are pharmacologically exactly the same. The color and packaging of pills dispensed in clinics may differ from pills in pharmacies.

The "ACHES" method of teaching women on pills what to watch out for and the problems a clinician or counselor should think about if one of these symptoms develops.

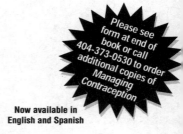

Please see form at end of book or call 404-373-0530 to order additional copies of Managing Contraception

Now available in English and Spanish

PROGESTIN - ONLY PILLS

**MICRONOR® TABLETS
28-DAY REGIMEN**
(0.35 mg norethindrone) (lime green)
Ortho-McNeil

=

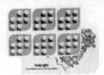

NOR-QD® TABLETS
(0.35 mg norethindrone) (yellow)
Watson

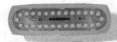

OVRETTE® TABLETS
(0.075 mg norgestrel) (yellow)
Wyeth-Ayerst

COMBINED PILLS - 20 microgram PILLS

ALESSE - 28 TABLETS
(0.1 mg levonorgestrel/20 mcg ethinyl estradiol)
(active pills pink)
Wyeth-Ayerst

=

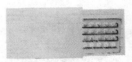

LEVLITE™ - 28 TABLETS
(0.1 mg levonorgestrel/20 mcg ethinyl estradiol)
(active pills pink)
Berlex

LOESTRIN® FE 1/20
(1 mg norethindrone acetate/20 mcg ethinyl
estradiol/75 mg ferrous fumarate [7d])
(active pills white)
Parke-Davis

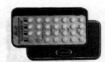

MIRCETTE - 28 TABLETS
(0.15 mg desogestrel/ 20 mcg ethinyl estradiol X 21 (white)/
placebo X 2 (green)/10 mcg ethinyl estradiol X 5 (yellow)
Organon

A15

COMBINED PILLS - 30 microgram PILLS

LEVLEN® 28 TABLETS
(0.15 mg levonorgestrel/30 mcg ethinyl estradiol)
(active pills light orange)
Berlex

=

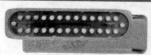

LO/OVRAL®-28 TABLETS
(0.3 mg norgestrel/30 mcg ethinyl estradiol)
(active pills white)
Wyeth-Ayerst

=

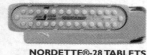

NORDETTE®-28 TABLETS
(0.15 mg levonorgestrel/30 mcg estradiol)
(active pills light orange)
Monarch

=

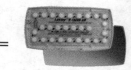

LEVORA TABLETS
(0.15 mg levonorgestrel/30 mcg ethinyl estradiol)
(active pills white)
Watson

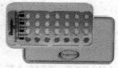

DESOGEN® 28 TABLETS
(0.15 mg desogestrel/30 mcg ethinyl estradiol)
(active pills white)
Organon

=

**ORTHO-CEPT® TABLETS
28-DAY REGIMEN**
(0.15 mg desogestrel/30 mcg ethinyl estradiol)
(active pills orange)
Ortho-McNeil

=

APRI

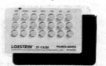

LOESTRIN® 21 1.5/30
(1.5 mg norethindrone acetate/ 30 mcg ethinyl estradiol)
(active pills green)
Parke-Davis

A16

COMBINED PILLS - 35 microgram PILLS

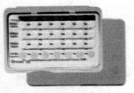

OVCON® 35 28-DAY
(0.4 mg norethindrone/35 mcg ethinyl estradiol)
(active pills peach)
Bristol-Myers

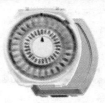

**ORTHO-CYCLEN®
28 TABLETS**
(0.25 mg norgestimate/35 mcg ethinyl estradiol)
(active pills blue)
Ortho-McNeil

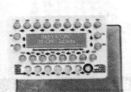

**BREVICON®
28-DAY TABLETS**
Also available:
BREVICON® 21-DAY TABLETS
(0.5 mg norethindrone/35 mcg ethinyl estradiol)
(active pills blue)
Watson

=

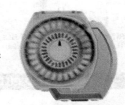

**MODICON® TABLETS
28-DAY REGIMEN**
(0.5 mg norethindrone/35 mcg ethinyl estradiol)
(active pills white)
Ortho-McNeil

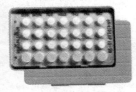

DEMULEN® 1/35-28
(1 mg ethynodiol diacetate/35 mcg ethinyl estradiol)
(active pills white)
Pharmacia

=

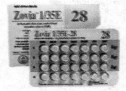

ZOVIA® 1/35E–28
(1 mg ethynodiol diacetate/35 mcg ethinyl estradiol)
(active pills light pink)
Watson

A17

COMBINED PILLS - 35 microgram PILLS (continued)

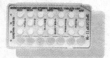 =

NORETHIN 1/35E–28
(1 mg norethindrone/35 mcg ethinyl estradiol)
(active pills white)
Shire

**ORTHO-NOVUM® 1/35
28 TABLETS**
(1 mg norethindrone/35 mcg ethinyl estradiol)
(active pills peach)
Ortho-McNeil

 =

NORINYL® 1+35 28-DAY TABLETS
(1 mg norethindrone/35 mcg ethinyl estradiol)
(active pills yellow-green)
Watson

NECON 1/35-28
(1 mg norethindrone/35 mcg ethinyl estradiol)
(active pills dark yellow)
Watson

COMBINED PILLS - PHASIC PILLS

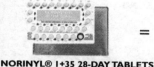 =

TRIPHASIL®-28 TABLETS
(levonorgestrel/ethinyl estradiol–triphasic regimen)
0.050 mg/30 mcg (6d) (brown),
0.075 mg/40 mcg (5d) (white),
0.125 mg/30 mcg (10d) (light yellow)
Wyeth-Ayerst

TRI-LEVLEN® 28 TABLETS
(levonorgestrel/ethinyl estradiol–triphasic regimen)
0.050 mg/30 mcg (6d) (brown),
0.075 mg/40 mcg (5d) (white),
0.125 mg/30 mcg (10d) (light yellow)
Berlex

TRIVORA®
(levonorgestrel/ethinyl estradiol–triphasic regimen)
0.050 mg/30 mcg (6d), 0.075 mg/40 mcg (5d),
0.125 mg/30 mcg (10d) (pink)
Watson

CYCLESSA
(desogestrel/ethinyl estradiol–triphasic regimen)
0. mg/25 mcg (7d) (light yellow)
0.125 mg/25 mcg (7d) (orange)
0.150 mg/25 mcg (7d) (red)
Organon

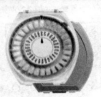

**ORTHO-NOVUM® 10/11
28 TABLETS**
(norethindrone/ethinyl estradiol)
0.5 mg/35 mcg (10d) (white),
1 mg/35 mcg (11d) (peach)
Ortho-McNeil

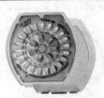

JENEST 28 TABLETS
(norethindrone/ethinyl estradiol)
0.5 mg/35 mcg (7d) (white),
1 mg/35 mcg (14d) (peach)
Organon

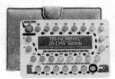

**TRI-NORINYL®
28-DAY TABLETS**
(norethindrone/ethinyl estradiol)
0.5 mg/35 mcg (7d) (blue),
1 mg/35 mcg (9d) (yellow-green),
0.5 mg/35 mcg (5d) (blue)
Watson

**ORTHO-NOVUM® 7/7/7
28 TABLETS**
(norethindrone/ethinyl estradiol)
0.5 mg/35 mcg (7d) (white),
0.75 mg/35 mcg (7d) (light peach),
1 mg/35 mcg (7d) (peach)
Ortho-McNeil

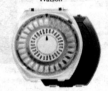

**ORTHO TRI-CYCLEN®
28 TABLETS**
(norgestimate/ethinyl estradiol)
0.18 mg/35 mcg (7d) (white),
0.215 mg/35 mcg (7d) (light blue),
0.25 mg/35 mcg (7d) (blue)
Ortho-McNeil

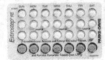

**ESTROSTEP® FE
28 TABLETS**
(norethindrone acetate/ethinyl estradiol)
1 mg/20 mcg (5d) (white triangular),
1 mg/30 mcg (7d) (white square),
1 mg/35 mcg (9d), 75 mg ferrous fumarate (7d)
(white round)
Parke-Davis

A19

COMBINED PILLS - 50 microgram PILLS

Pills with 50 micrograms of mestranol are not as strong as pills with 50 micrograms of ethinyl estradiol

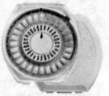

**ORTHO-NOVUM® 1/50
28 TABLETS**
(1 mg norethindrone/50 mcg mestranol)
(active pills yellow)
Ortho-McNeil

=

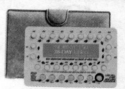

**NORINYL® 1+50
28-DAY TABLETS**
(1 mg norethindrone/50 mcg mestranol)
(active pills white)
Watson

||

**NECON 1/50
28-DAY TABLETS**
(1 mg norethindrone/50 mcg mestranol)
Watson

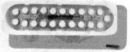

OVRAL - 21 TABLETS
(0.5 mg norgestrel/50 mcg ethinyl estradiol)
(active pills white)
Wyeth-Ayerst

=

OGESTREL
Watson

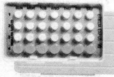

DEMULEN® 1/50-28
(1 mg ethynodiol diacetate/50 mcg ethinyl estradiol)
(active pills white)
Watson

||

ZOVIA® 1/50E-21 and 28
(1 mg ethynodiol diacetate/50 mcg ethinyl estradiol)
Watson

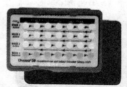

OVCON® 50 28-DAY
(1 mg norethindrone/50 mcg ethinyl estradiol)
(active pills yellow)
Warner-Chilcott

A20

PILL WARNING SIGNALS

Pills have been studied extensively and are very safe. However, very rarely pills lead to serious problems. Here are the warning signals to watch out for while using pills. These warning signals spell out the word **ACHES**. If you have one of these symptoms, it may or may not be related to pill use. You need to check with your clinician as soon as possible. The problems that could possibly be related to using pills are as follows:

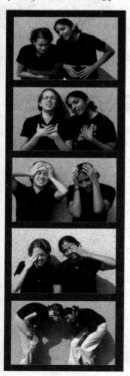

ABDOMINAL PAIN
- Blood clot in the pelvis or liver
- Benign liver tumor or gall bladder disease

CHEST PAIN
- Blood clot in the lungs
- Heart attack
- Angina (heart pain)
- Breast lump

HEADACHES
- Stroke
- Migraine headache with neurological problems (blurred vision, spots, zigzag lines, weakness, difficulty speaking)
- Other headaches caused by pills
- High blood pressure

EYE PROBLEMS
- Stroke
- Blurred vision, double vision, or loss of vision
- Migraine headache with neurological problems (blurred vision, spots, zigzag lines)
- Blood clots in the eyes
- Change in shape of cornea (contacts don't fit)

SEVERE LEG PAIN
- Inflammation and blood clots of a vein in the leg

You should also return to the office if you develop severe mood swings or depression, become jaundiced (yellow-colored skin), miss 2 periods or have signs of pregnancy.

PILLS AS EMERGENCY CONTRACEPTIVES:

2 Different Approaches: Combined Pills OR Progestin-Only Pills

PROGESTIN-ONLY PILLS

1 + 1 pill 12 hours apart

Plan B

20 + 20 pills 12 hours apart

Ovrette *(yellow pills)*

(Plan B and Ovrette are NOT carried
in all pharmacies. Check in advance.)

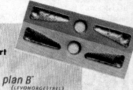

plan B®
(LEVONORGESTREL)

PLAN B

COMBINED ORAL CONTRACEPTIVES

2 + 2 pills 12 hours apart

Preven *(blue pills)* OR
Ogestrel *(white pills)* OR
Ovral *(white pills)*

(Preven Ogestrel and Ovral are NOT carried
in all pharmacies. Check in advance.)

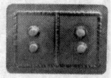

PREVEN

4 + 4 pills 12 hours apart

Low-Ogestrel *(white pills)*
Lo-Ovral *(white pills)*,
Levora *(white pills)* OR
Levlen *(light orange pills)* OR
Nordette *(light orange pills)* OR
Triphasil *(yellow pills)*,
Tri-Levlen *(yellow pills)* OR
Trivora *(pink pills)*

5 + 5 pills 12 hours apart

Alesse *(pink pills)* OR Levlite *(pink pills)*